The Awful T

CHEMOTHERAPY & RADIATION

CANCER RESEARCH INTERNATIONAL
Report on Chemotherapy & Radiation
CancersAnswers.org

MEDICAL PROFESSION: No other profession charges as much and accomplishes as little.

EXCERPT FROM CANCERS ANSWERS

VOLUME 1 + PAGE 161

CANCERSANSWERS.ORG

Cancer drugs aren't just really expensive; they're a bad value

BY CAROLYN JOHNSON

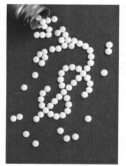

With some cancer drug prices soaring past $10,000 a month, doctors have begun to ask one nagging question:

Do drug prices correctly reflect the value they bring to patients by extending or improving their lives?

A study published Thursday in JAMA Oncology aims to answer that question by examining necitumumab, an experimental lung cancer drug made by Eli Lilly & Co.

The drug isn't approved yet and Eli Lilly has not set a price. However, there is data on how well it works: in a clinical trial, researchers found that adding the drug to chemotherapy extended life by 1.6 months, on average, for patients with a dire prognosis — a type of non-small cell lung cancer that has spread.

In order to estimate what the price of this drug *should* be, based on its value to patients, the research team modeled various scenarios. Generally, economists suggest that one additional year in perfect health in the U.S. is worth somewhere between $50,000 and $200,000 a year. Although some patients taking *necitumumab* lived a little longer, people with advanced cancer often have a lower quality of life than healthy people and the researchers took that into consideration.

Based on their calculations, the drug should cost from $563 to $1,309 for a three-week cycle.

That is much lower than the typical new cancer drug, which can cost patients many thousands of dollars per month.

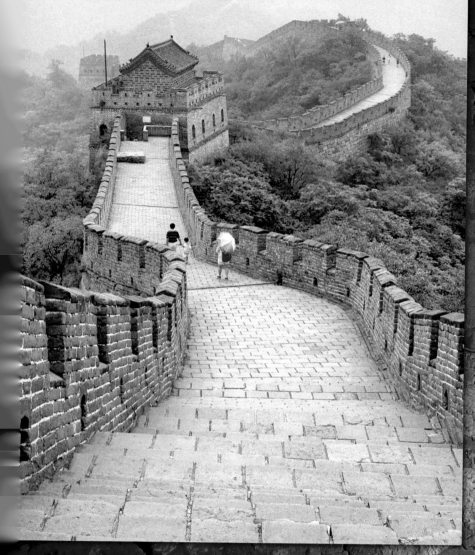

You cannot know ways you have not traveled.

EXCERPT FROM **CANCERS ANSWERS**

VOLUME 1 + PAGE 289
CANCERSANSWERS.ORG

"Currently, the prices of cancer drugs are increasing and the prices are not linked to the benefit that the drug provides," Daniel Goldstein, an oncologist at the Winship Cancer Institute at Emory University who led the study, said in an email.

"We propose that drugs that provide a minimal benefit should have a lower price, while drugs that provide a major benefit should have a higher price. Ideally, this method of value based pricing should financially incentivize researchers and industry to develop truly game-changing innovations."

A spokeswoman for Eli Lilly said that the design of the study was sound, but had some obvious limitations, including the types of drugs the researchers compared to *necitumumab*. "The pricing of cancer medicines is complex, and Lilly recognizes that assessing value is extraordinarily difficult," spokeswoman Crystal Livers-Powers said in an email.

"It is premature to discuss the drug's price," she said.

"Squamous non-small cell lung cancer that has spread," Livers-Powers said, "is a devastating, difficult-to-treat disease with a high unmet medical need."

Goldstein and his collaborators have done this kind of analysis before. They found, for example, that the price of the advanced colon cancer drug, *regorafenib*, assumes that the value of an additional year of life in perfect health is more than $700,000 — more than three times what most economists suggest we should be paying. The price of *bevacizumab* for advanced colon cancer reflects a year of life valued somewhere between $350,000 and $500,000, but those drugs are already on the market, and prices that are already set can be hard to budge. The researchers said they decided to do this study because the Food and Drug Administration is expected to make a decision on whether the company can sell the drug by year's end. So, they hope their analysis of the value might factor into the price, if it gains approval.

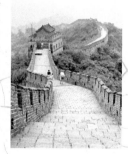

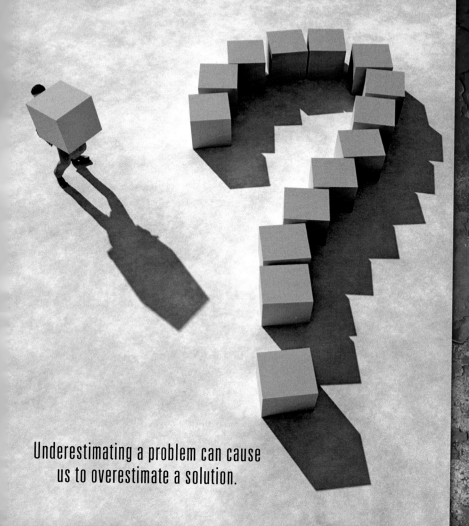

Underestimating a problem can cause
us to overestimate a solution.

EXCERPT FROM CANCERS ANSWERS

VOLUME 1 + PAGE 116
CANCERSANSWERS.ORG

Another recent study by researchers at the University of Texas MD Anderson Cancer Center found that treatments for many blood cancers were overpriced compared to their value. In the journal *Cancer*, those researchers examined two dozen studies and found that the cost of extended healthy life provided by these drugs exceeded $50,000 a year. In some cases, the drugs were priced to reflect an additional year of life valued between $210,000 to $426,000 — well above what economists think we should pay.

PhRMA, a trade group for the drug industry, defended the industry's pricing practices, noting that cancer drug costs represent just a fifth of total cancer care spending.

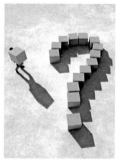

There are many variables that go into the price of a drug, but mounting evidence suggests that the value it brings to patients is not the biggest factor.

"How they price the drug is by pricing it at whatever the market is wiling to bear," said Benjamn Djulbegovic, an oncologist at the University of South Florida.

http://www.washingtonpost.com/news/wonkblog/wp/2015/08/27/cancer-drugs-arent-just-really-expensive-theyre-a-bad-value/

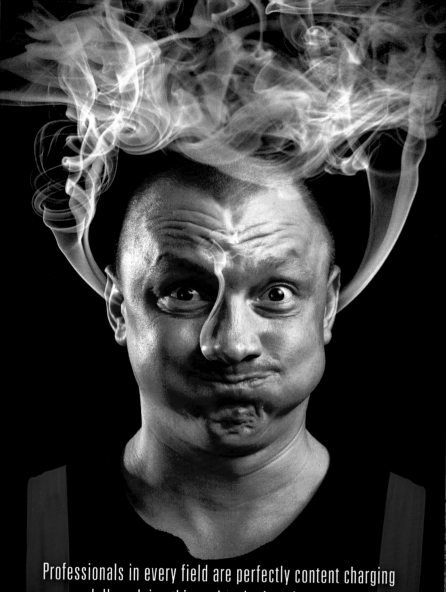

Professionals in every field are perfectly content charging
dollars doing things that don't make sense.

EXCERPT FROM CANCERS ANSWERS

VOLUME 1 + PAGE 181
CANCERSANSWERS.ORG

60 MINUTES

"The Cost of Cancer Drugs"

AIRED ON OCT. 5, 2014

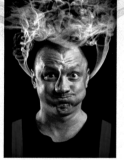

Cancer is so pervasive that it touches virtually every family in this country. More than one out of three Americans will be diagnosed with some form of cancer in their lifetime. And as anyone who's been through it knows, the shock and anxiety of the diagnosis is followed by a second jolt: the high price of all cancer drugs.

They are so astronomical that a growing number of patients can't afford their co-pay, the percentage of their drug bill they have to pay out-of-pocket.

This has led to a revolt against the drug companies led by some of the most prominent cancer doctors in the country.

Dr. Leonard Saltz: We're in a situation where a cancer diagnosis is one of the leading causes of personal bankruptcy.

Dr. Leonard Saltz is chief of gastrointestinal oncology at Memorial Sloan Kettering, one of the nation's premier cancer centers, and he's a leading expert on colon cancer.

Lesley Stahl: So, are you saying in effect, that we have to start treating the cost of these drugs almost like a side effect from cancer?

Dr. Leonard Saltz: I think that's a fair way of looking at it. We're starting to see the term *financial toxicity* being used in the literature. Individual patients are going into bankruptcy trying to deal with these prices.

I do worry that people's fear and anxiety's are being taken advantage of.

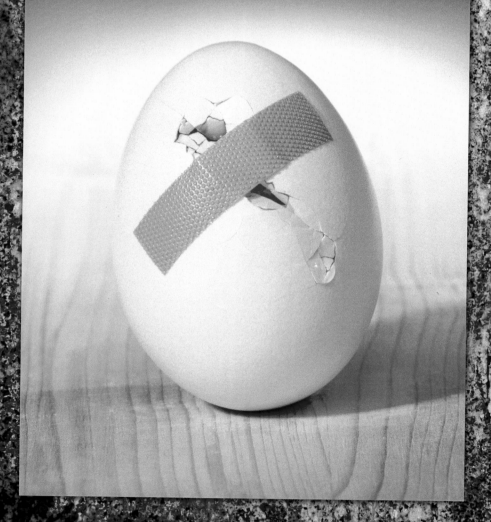

How can anyone improve your health
by unnecessarily damaging your body?

EXCERPT FROM CANCERS ANSWERS

VOLUME 1 + PAGE 173
CANCERSANSWERS.ORG

Lesley Stahl: The general price for a new drug is what?

Dr. Leonard Saltz: They're priced at well over $100,000 a year.

Lesley Stahl: Wow.

Dr. Leonard Saltz: And remember that many of these drugs, most of them, don't replace everything else. They get added to it. And if you figure one drug costs $120,000 and the next drug's not going to cost less, you're at a quarter-million dollars in drug costs just to get started.

Lesley Stahl: I mean, you're dealing with people who are desperate.

Dr. Leonard Saltz: I do worry that people's fear and anxiety are being taken advantage of. And yes, it costs money to develop these drugs, but I do think the price is too high.

The drug companies say it costs over a billion dollars to bring a new drug to market, so the prices reflect the cost of innovation.

So many in the middle class struggle to meet the cost of their co-payments. Sometimes they take half-doses of the drug to save money. Or delay getting their prescriptions refilled.

Dr. Saltz's battle against the cost of cancer drugs started in 2012 when the FDA approved *Zaltrap* for treating advanced colon cancer. Saltz compared the clinical trial results of Zaltrap to those of another drug already on the market, *Avastin*. He says both target the same patient population, work essentially in the same way. And, when given as part of chemotherapy, deliver the identical result: extending median survival by 1.4 months, or 42 days.

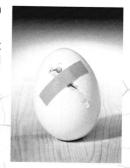

Dr. Leonard Saltz: They looked to be about the same. To me, it locked like a Coke and Pepsi sort of thing.

Then Saltz, as head of the hospital's pharmacy committee, discovered how much it would cost: roughly $11,000 per month, more than twice that of Avastin.

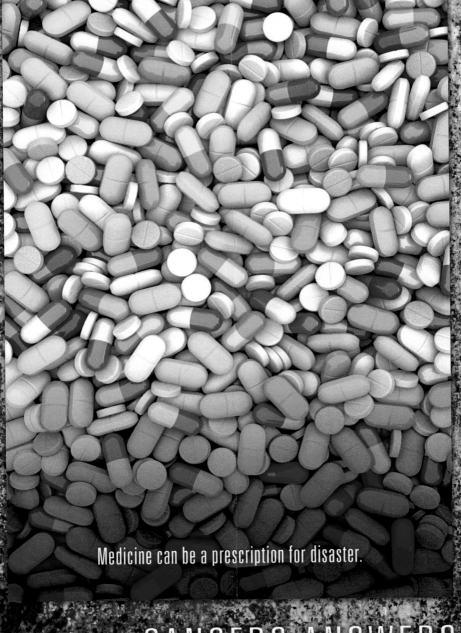

Medicine can be a prescription for disaster.

EXCERPT FROM CANCERS ANSWERS

VOLUME 1 + PAGE 105
CANCERSANSWERS.ORG

The Eye Popping Cost of Cancer Drugs

Lesley Stahl: So $5,000 versus $11,000. That's quite a jump. Did it have fewer side effects? Was it less toxic? Did it have…

Dr. Leonard Saltz: No…

Lesley Stahl: …Something that would have explained this double price?

Dr. Leonard Saltz: If anything, it looked like there might be a little more toxicity in the Zaltrap study.

He contacted Dr. Peter Bach, Sloan Kettering's in-house expert on cancer drug prices.

Lesley Stahl: So Zaltrap. One day your phone rings and it's Dr. Saltz. Do you remember what he said?

Dr. Peter Bach: He said, "Peter, I think we're not going to include a new cancer drug because it costs too much."

Lesley Stahl: Had you ever heard a line like that before?

Dr. Peter Bach: No. My response was, "I'll be right down."

Lesley Stahl: You ran down.

Dr. Peter Bach: I think I took the elevator. But yes, exactly.

Bach determined that since patients would have to take Zaltrap for several months, the price tag for 42 days of extra life would run to nearly $60,000. What they then decided to do was unprecedented: reject a drug just because of its price.

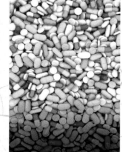

Dr. Peter Bach: We did it for one reason. Because we need to take into account the financial consequences of the decisions that we make for our patients. Patients in Medicare would pay more than $2,000 a month themselves, out-of-pocket, for Zaltrap. And that was the same as the typical income every month for a patient in Medicare.

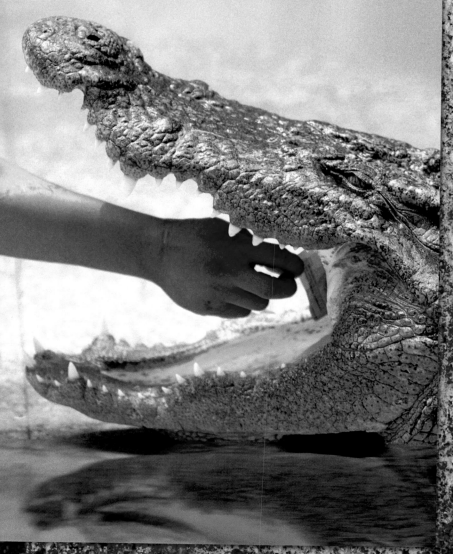

Don't try things out that can do you in.

EXCERPT FROM CANCERS ANSWERS

VOLUME 1 • PAGE 109

CANCERSANSWERS.ORG

Lesley Stahl: The co-pay.

Dr. Peter Bach: Right. 20 percent. Taking money from their children's inheritance, from the money they've saved. We couldn't in good conscience say, we're going to prescribe this more expensive drug.

It was a shocking event. Because it was irrefutable evidence that the price was a falsehood.

And, then they proclaimed their decision in the New York Times, blasting what they called *runaway cancer drug prices*. It was a shot across the bow of the pharmaceutical industry and Congress for passing laws that Bach says allow the drug companies to charge whatever they want for cancer medications.

Dr. Peter Bach: Medicare has to pay exactly what the drug company charges. Whatever that number is.

Lesley Stahl: Wait a minute, this is a law?

Dr. Peter Bach: Yes.

Lesley Stahl: And there's no negotiating whatsoever with Medicare?

Dr. Peter Bach: No.

Another reason drug prices are so expensive, according to an independent study, is that the single biggest source of income for private practice oncologists is their "commission" from cancer drugs (chemotherapy & radiation). **They buy the drugs wholesale from the pharmaceutical companies, they set the retail price, and they sell them retail to their patients.**

Dr. Leonard Saltz: What that does is create a very substantial incentive to use a more expensive drug, because if you're getting a percent of $10, that's nothing. If you're getting percent of $10,000, or $100,000 that starts to mount up. So, now you have a real conflict of interest that translates into bias and prejudice, influencing what they recommend and it all starts with the drug companies setting the wholesale price (Doctor's cost).

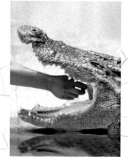

Dr. Peter Bach: We have a pricing system for drugs which is completely dictated by the people who are making the drugs.

Doctors rarely miss an opportunity
to miss a diagnosis.

EXCERPT FROM CANCERS ANSWERS

VOLUME 1 • PAGE 103

CANCERSANSWERS.ORG

Lesley Stahl: How do you think they're deciding the price?

Dr. Peter Bach: It's corporate chutzpah (whatever they can get away with).

Lesley Stahl: We'll just raise the price, period.

Dr. Peter Bach: Just a question of how brave they are and how little they want to end up in the New York Times or on 60 Minutes.

That's because media exposure, he says, works. Right after their editorial was published, the drug's manufacturer, Sanofi, cut the price of Zaltrap by more than half.

Dr. Peter Bach: It was a shocking event. Because it was irrefutable evidence that the price was a falsehood. All of those arguments that we've heard for decades: we have to charge the price we charge; we have to recoup our money; we're good for society; trust us; we'll set the right price. One op-ed in the New York Times quoted one hospital as saying, "Oh, okay, we'll charge a different price." It was like we were negotiating at a Turkish bazaar.

Lesley Stahl: What do you mean?

Dr. Peter Bach: They said, "This carpet is $500 and you say, "I'll give you $100." And the guy says, "Okay." They set it up to make it highly profitable for doctors to go for Zaltrap instead of Avastin. It was crazy!

But, he says it got even crazier when Sanofi explained the way they were changing the price.

Dr. Peter Bach: They lowered it in a way that doctors could get the drug for less, but patients were still paying as if it was high-priced.

Lesley Stahl: Oh, come on.

Dr. Peter Bach: They said to the doctor, buy Zaltrap from us for $11,000 and we'll send you a check for $6,000. Then you give it to your patient and you get to bill the patient's insurance company as if it cost $11,000. So it made it extremely profitable for the doctors. They could basically double their money when they pick Zaltrap to use.

Real knowledge is to know the extent of one's ignorance.
                                                              - Confucius

0

Interpretations are often different from reality.

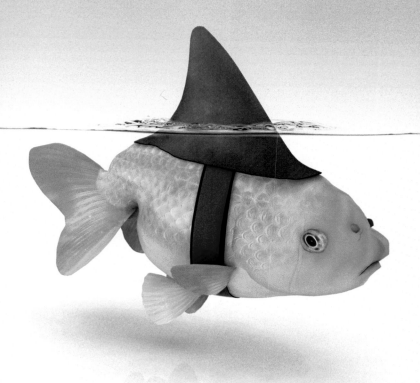

EXCERPT FROM CANCERS ANSWERS

VOLUME 1 + PAGE 339

CANCERSANSWERS.ORG

Lesley Stahl: If you are taking a drug that's no better than another drug already on the market and charging twice as much, and everybody thought the original drug was too much. All this is now accepted industry practice.

John Castellani: We don't set the prices on what the patient pays. What a patient pays is determined by his or her insurance.

Lesley Stahl: Are you saying that the pharmaceutical company's not to blame for how much the patient is paying? You're saying it's the insurance company?

John Castellani: I'm saying the insurance model makes the medicine seem artificially expensive for the patient.

He's talking about the high co-pay for cancer drugs. If you're on Medicare, you pay 20 percent.

Lesley Stahl: Twenty percent of $11,000 a month is a heck of a lot more than 20 percent of $5,000 a month.

John Castellani: But why should it be 20 percent instead of five percent?

Lesley Stahl: Why should it be $11,000 a month?

John Castellani: Because the cost of developing these therapies is so expensive.

Lesley Stahl: Then why did Sanofi cut it in half when they got some bad publicity?

John Castellani: I can't respond to a specific company.

Sanofi declined our request for an interview, but said in this email that they lowered the price of Zaltrap after listening "to early feedback from the oncology community (they used to call this *getting caught*) and... To ensure affordable choices for patients...

Dr. Hagop Kantarjian: High cancer drug prices are harming patients because either you come up with the money, or you die.

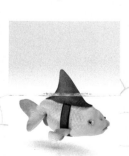

Hagop Kantarjian chairs the department of leukemia at MD Anderson in Houston. Inspired by the doctors at Sloan Kettering, he enlisted 119 of the world's leading leukemia specialists to cosign this article about the high price of drugs that don't just add a few weeks of life, but actually add years, like Gleevec.

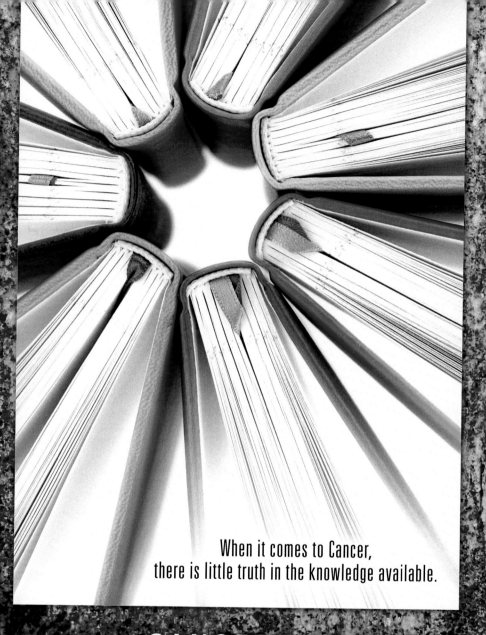

When it comes to Cancer,
there is little truth in the knowledge available.

EXCERPT FROM CANCERS ANSWERS
VOLUME 1 • PAGE 33
CANCERSANSWERS.ORG

Nat'l Oncologists Group Tackles Spiraling Drug Costs

It treats CML, one of the most common types of blood cancers that used to be a death sentence, but with Gleevec most patients survive for 10 years or more.

Dr. Hagop Kantarjian: This is probably the best drug we ever developed in cancer.

Lesley Stahl: In all cancers?

Dr. Hagop Kantarjian: So far. And that shows the dilemma, because here you have a drug that makes people live their normal life. But, in order to live normally, they are enslaved by the cost of the drug. They have to pay every year for the rest of their life.

Lesley Stahl: You have to stay on it. You have to keep taking it.

Dr. Hagop Kantarjian: You have to stay on it indefinitely. Gleevec is the top selling drug for industry giant Novartis, bringing in more than $4 billion a year in sales. $35 billion since the drug came to market. There are now several other drugs like it. So, you'd think with the competition, the price of Gleevec would have come down.

Dr. Hagop Kantarjian: And yet, the price of the drug tripled from $28,000 a year in 2001 to $92,000 a year in 2012.

They are making prices unreasonable, unsustainable and, in my opinion, immoral.

Lesley Stahl: Are you saying that the drug companies are raising the prices on their older drugs.

Dr. Hagop Kantarjian: That's correct.

Lesley Stahl: Not just the new ones. So, you have a new drug that might come out at a $100,000, but they are also saying the old drugs have to come up to that price, too?

Dr. Hagop Kantarjian: Exactly. They are making prices unreasonable, unsustainable and, in my opinion, immoral.

When we asked Novartis why they tripled the price of Gleevec, they told us, "Gleevec has been a life-changing medicine ... When setting the prices of our medicines we consider ... the benefits they bring to patients ... The price of existing treatments and the investments needed to continue to innovate..."

[Dr. Hagop Kantarjian: This is quite an expensive medication.]

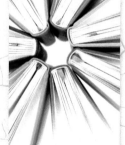

S

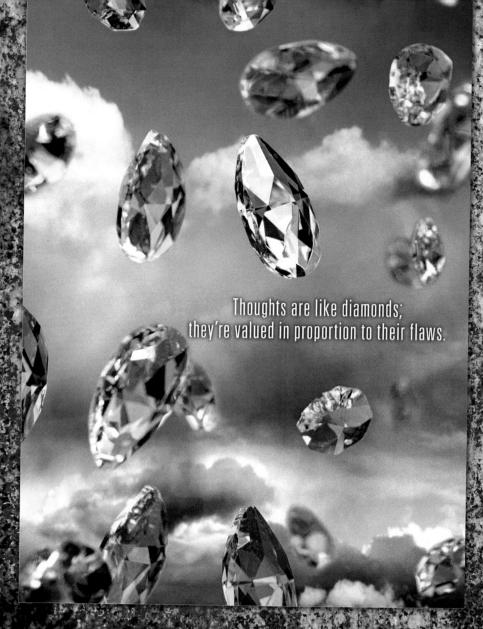

Thoughts are like diamonds;
they're valued in proportion to their flaws.

EXCERPT FROM CANCERS ANSWERS

VOLUME 1 + PAGE 230
CANCERSANSWERS.ORG

Dr. Kantarjian says one thing that has to change is the law that prevents Medicare from negotiating for lower prices.

Dr. Hagop Kantarjian: This is unique to the United States. If you look anywhere in the world, there are negotiations. Either by the government or by different regulatory bodies to regulate the price of the drug. And this is why the prices are 50 percent to 80 percent lower anywhere in the world compared to the United States.

Lesley Stahl: Fifty percent to 80 percent?

Dr. Hagop Kantarjian: Fifty percent to 80 percent.

Lesley Stahl: The same drug?

Dr. Hagop Kantarjian: Same drug. American patients end up paying two to three times more for the same drug compared to Canadians or Europeans or Australians and others.

Lesley Stahl: Now, Novartis, which makes Gleevec, says that the price is fair because this is a miracle drug. It really works.

Dr. Hagop Kantarjian: The only drug that works is a drug that a patient can afford.

The challenge, Dr. Saltz at Sloan Kettering says, is knowing where to draw the line between how long a drug extends life and how much it costs.

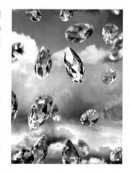

Lesley Stahl: Where is that line?

Dr. Leonard Saltz: I don't know where that line is, but we as a society have been unwilling to discuss this topic and, as a result, the only people that are setting the line are the people that are selling the drugs.

Source: http://www.cbsnews.com/news/the-cost-of-cancer-drugs/

He who asks is a fool for five minutes, but he who does not ask remains a fool forever.

- Chinese proverb

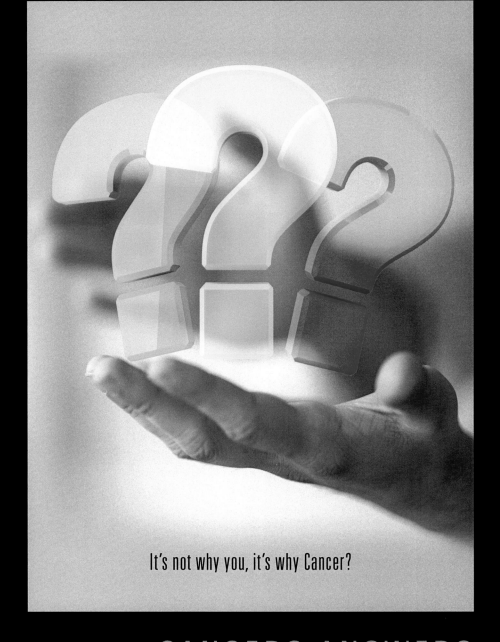

It's not why you, it's why Cancer?

EXCERPT FROM CANCERS ANSWERS

VOLUME 1 + PAGE 17

CANCERSANSWERS.ORG

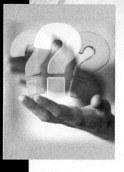

TABLE**CONTENTS**

You need to battle Cancer,
not the treatments.

EXCERPT FROM CANCERS ANSWERS
VOLUME 1 ✦ PAGE 31
CANCERSANSWERS.ORG

what IS CHEMOTHERAPY?

Third among the so-called medically proven methods of *treating* cancer is toxic chemotherapy (the other two being surgery and radiation): the use of strong, toxic drugs to try to kill cancer cells. Few topics in medicine today are as controversial as the use of these toxic agents, and for good factual reasons.

"In theory, a drug cure for cancer is highly appealing as we have all been conditioned to believe there is a *doctor* and a *pill* for everything. Just as specific drugs *seem to cure* many bacterial and parasitic infections, we want to believe chemotherapy should ideally kill cancer cells without harming excessive numbers of normal cells, tissues, and organs. In reality, however, chemotherapy has not yet developed an agent specific enough, and safe enough, to limit its attack and destruction to cancer cells only. Many chemotherapeutic agents work by blocking an essential metabolic step in the process of cellular division. Since cancer cells often divide more rapidly than normal cells, this lethal anti-metabolite action should be directed preferentially against cancer cells, only. However, most normal tissues of the body engage in cell division at different rates. Thus, chemotherapy poisons vast amounts of normal cells, tissues, organs, and systems of the body as well, and at the same time, especially the rapidly dividing cells of the bone marrow, intestinal wall (a big percent of your immune system) and hair follicles, etc." says Dr. Ralph Moss.[2]

[1] Morgan, G., Ward, R., and Barton, M. PubMed.gov. from *Clinical Oncology (R Coll Radioll)* 2004, Dec; 16(8):549-60

[2] Moss, Ralph W. *The Cancer Industry.* Page 74. State College, PA, 1999, 2002. Wikipedia. http://en.wikipedia.org/wiki/Chemotherapy

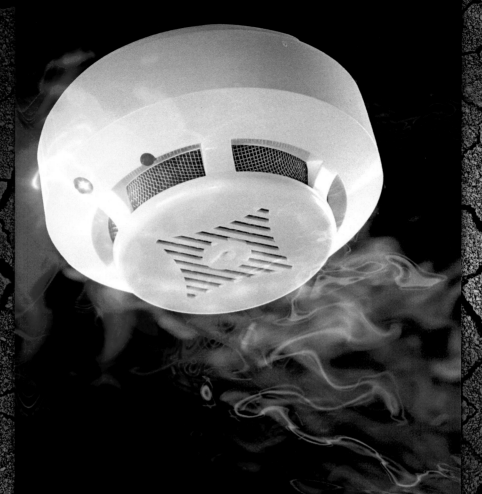

Awareness of symptoms is like a smoke detector,
it only goes off after the fire has started.

EXCERPT FROM CANCERS ANSWERS

VOLUME 1 + PAGE 548
CANCERSANSWERS.ORG

IS CHEMOTHERAPY?

The bone marrow is, of course, the foundation of the immune system, which seems to serve the dual function of preventing infections and combating the spread of infectious cancer. The use of chemotherapy is accompanied by inherent destruction of the immune system, and often brings with it a host of other blood deficiency diseases including leukopenia, thrombocytopenia, aplastic anemia, and many others, some of which are worse than the cancer you started with. These, in turn, can give rise to massive, uncontrollable infections (underlying Primary "causes" of cancer). **Cancer patients on chemotherapy have been known to die of something as innocuous as the common cold.**[3]

Chemotherapy's effect on the gut can be equally disastrous. Cancer patients sometimes have difficulty eating, digesting, or

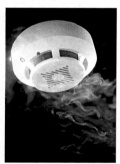 absorbing and assimilating their food and nutrients. Cancer drugs cause extreme nausea, bleeding sores around the mouth and throughout the insides, soreness of the gums and throat, and ulceration and bleeding of the gastrointestinal tract, because the mucous cells are rapid dividers, chemotherapy can result in the entire sloughing of the internal mucosa of the gut, which can lead to death. [4, 5]

[3] Ibid.

[4] Ibid.

[5] Moss, Ralph W. *The Cancer Industry*. Page 74. State College, PA, 1999, 2002.

PART I: Why Chemotherapy Does Not Work 97.9% of the Time[1]

The worst symptoms from disease
can be from treatments for it.

EXCERPT FROM

CANCERS ANSWERS

VOLUME 1 ✦ PAGE 40

CANCERSANSWERS.ORG

CHEMOTHERAPY IS toxic

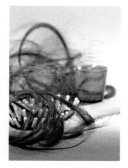

All chemotherapy drugs have one thing in common: **they are *poisonous*.** The little they seem to work is directly because they're poisonous. This is a concentrated effort to kill the cancer before killing the patient. It often does not work that way and **patients statistically do die from every known chemotherapy agent in current use, often far earlier** than the cancer would have done so, but not before massive negative reactions. Methotrexate, for example, carries with it the following warning:[6]

ONLY PHYSICIANS EXPERIENCED IN ANTIMETABOLITE CHEMOTHERAPY MUST USE METHOTREXATE.

BECAUSE THE POSSIBILITY OF FATAL OR SEVERE TOXIC REACTIONS, THE PATIENT SHOULD BE FULLY INFORMED BY THE PHYSICIAN OF THE RISKS INVOLVED AND SHOULD BE UNDER HIS CONSTANT SUPERVISION.

(Physician's Desk Reference)

The package insert goes on to describe the ***high potential toxicity*** of the product. This includes the above-mentioned symptoms and adds malaise, undue fatigue, chills and fever, dizziness, and various problems with skin, blood, alimentary system, urogenital system, and central nervous system. Finally, the doctor is warned that:

Other reactions related or attributed to the use of methotrexate such as pneumonitis, metabolic changes, precipitating diabetes, osteoporotic effects, abnormal tissue, cell changes, and even sudden death have been reported.

---

[6] Ibid.

Medical treatments often do more "to you" than "for you."

CANCERS ANSWERS

VOLUME 1 ✦ PAGE 80
CANCERSANSWERS.ORG

devastating

SIDE EFFECTS

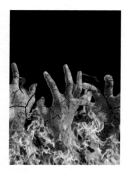

Dr. Laszlo, a former senior vice president at the American Cancer Institute and expert on the complications of cancer care cites that many patients suffer extreme nausea and vomiting, and that one-quarter of long-term patients will have these reactions even in the absence of these drugs. Dr. Ralph Moss confides that he has even heard doctors jokingly refer to the chemotherapy drugs 5-FU (*Five Feet Under*), and BCNU referred to as *Be Seein' You*. [7]

[7] Moss, Ralph W. *The Cancer Industry*. Pages 77-93. State College, PA, 1999, 2002.

Are you creating your problem
faster than you're solving it?

EXCERPT FROM CANCERS ANSWERS

VOLUME 1 ◆ PAGE 433

CANCERSANSWERS.ORG

chemotherapy
IS CARCINOGENIC [CAUSES CANCER]

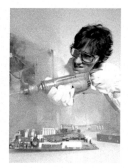

Another drawback to chemotherapy is the increased incidence of second malignancies, apparently what they call *unrelated* malignancies in patients who have been *cured* by means of anti-cancer drugs. This is probably because the drugs themselves are carcinogenic, and none of the current chemotherapy drugs can destroy the *stem cells* that cancer cells themselves produce. When chemotherapy and radiation are used in treatment, **secondary tumors occur at approximately 25 times the expected rate** according to the Cancer Institute of America.[8]

Since both chemotherapy and radiation treatment *suppress* the immune system, it is probable that new tumors are allowed to grow because the treatment(s) have rendered the patient unable to resist them. In either case, a person who is *cured* of cancer by these drastic means will find themselves struggling with a new drug induced tumor and other new side effects (illnesses) a few months, or a few years later.

---

[8] Benson, Jonathan. "Why chemotherapy doesn't work - Cancer tumors confirmed to have stem cells that regenerate tumors." *Natural News.com*, 2012

Using treatments for disease can be like
"rearranging your furniture on your Titanic."

disillusionment

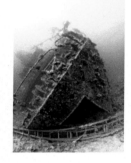

Even doctors sympathetic to chemotherapy and radiation admit that they have been near the limits of their utility for many years (Maugh and Marx, 1975). Any rational assessment of the efficacy of chemotherapy must be forced to include an admission that chemotherapy is only *rarely* curative in solid malignancies, particularly advanced solid malignancies and these rare ones still have the permanent damage from the treatment(s). Notable exceptions include testicular cancer (which is what Lance Armstrong was cured of) and anal cancer (an even bigger mess when it doesn't work). In contrast, "for hematological malignancies, such as leukemia and lymphoma, chemotherapy is usually the mainstay of doctor recommended therapy" writes super advocate for chemotherapy David Gorski (2011).[9]

There are literally hundreds of examples of chemotherapeutic drugs announced with great fanfare and promise, only to see them fall off of their lofty claims after initial reports are released. Dr. Ralph Moss writes in *The Cancer Industry* of literally dozens (the majority) of these promising, hopeful drug announcements and their failures over the last 60 years, a time when the initial interest and excitement began. **We literally have made almost no real progress in the long-term survival rate with chemotherapy since the 1950's.**[10] The drug companies literally re-formulate, re-name and re-package these drugs so the doctors will be able to hold out the *hope* of a *new* chemo drug and the illusion of a "new," false, toxic hope.

[9] Ibid.
[10] Ibid.

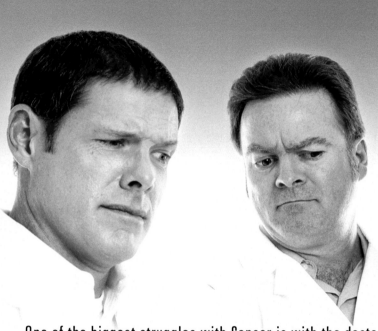

One of the biggest struggles with Cancer is with the doctors.

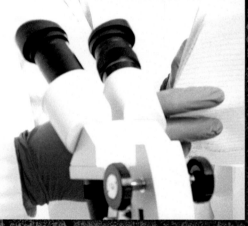

EXCERPT FROM CANCERS ANSWERS
VOLUME 1 + PAGE 180
CANCERSANSWERS.ORG

Even Charles Moertel, the Mayo Clinic researcher, famous for his negative tests of laetrile and vitamin C, charged that IL-2 was in fact **highly toxic, inordinately expensive, and not particularly effective** in an editorial in the *Journal of the American Medical Association.* "This specific treatment approach would not seem to merit further application of the *compassionate* management of patients with cancer," wrote Moertel. Commenting on the toxicity, "Treatment with IL-2 is an awesome experience. Patients require weeks of hospitalization in intensive care units if they are to survive the devastating toxic reactions of the chemotherapy alone. The dollar costs are six figures and the **benefits are questionable at best.**"[11]

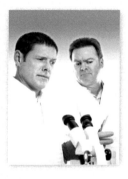

The initial report of his study showed remission in only 4% of patients, with the deaths during treatment of 16% of patients.[12] This means one would be trading the 16% likelihood of death for the 4% uncertainty of success with the 100% certainty of toxicity, toxic reactions, permanent damage to multiple parts of the body, lousy quality of life, the potential of death at any time from the treatment, and a guaranteed shorter life-span.

[11] Journal of the American Medical Association. *Science.* January 9, 1987. Moertel, C. G. "On Lymphokines, Cytokines, and Breakthroughs." Journal of America Medical Association 256:3141, 1986.

[12] *New York Times.* April 9, 1987.

PART I: Why Chemotherapy Does Not Work 97.9% of the Time[1]

The best treatments can make the causes worse.

EXCERPT FROM CANCERS ANSWERS

VOLUME 1 ✦ PAGE 390
CANCERSANSWERS.ORG

limited

SUCCESSES

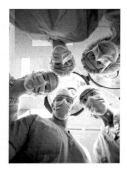

If these drugs were highly effective, one might tolerate their admittedly harsh side effects to get the benefit of a potential cure. They are not without a few successes either. A very few, and mostly very rare types of cancer are treated *successfully* with chemotherapy. The limited successes are limited to small tumors that have only recently developed (not recurrences). According to Marx and Maugh, chemotherapy is not very effective against tumors that have grown over time, existed for a long time, or metastasized. **Certainly, the big killer cancers, colon, breast, prostate and lung malignancies generally do not respond to chemotherapy at all.**[13]

Choriocarcinoma, a rare tumor in pregnant women is acknowledged to be effective in 75- 85% of cases according to the *Merck Manual*, 1987. Burkitt's Lymphoma has been successfully in approximately 50% of cases. This cancer is extremely rare in the U.S. and most cases are found only in Africa (Maugh and Marx, 1975).[14] Lymphoblastic leukemia in children has shown a 90% remission and 70% survival rate.[15] They all (survivors) have the same long-term result of damaged cells, tissues, organs and systems of the body, continued complications with normal functions of the body, greater tendency to easily develop other diseases, and shorter life-span.

[13] Moss, Ralph W. *The Cancer Industry*. Pages 77-93. State College, PA, 1999, 2002.

[14] *Merck Manual*, 1987.

[15] Maugh, Thomas H. and Marx, Jean L. *Seeds of Destruction: The Science Report of Cancer Research*. New York: Plenum Publishing Corporation, 1975.

Don't bet on "good" being enough.

EXCERPT FROM CANCERS ANSWERS

VOLUME 1 + PAGE 172
CANCERSANSWERS.ORG

Other forms of cancer that have shown some promise include acute lymphocytic leukemia, Ewing's sarcoma, neuroblastoma, osteogenic sarcoma, ovarian cancer, testicular cancer, and rhabdomyosarcoma. That is a *small group* with *limited* results. Let's try to put this into perspective. Everyone champions the very rare choriocarcinoma with therapeutic success. However, Dr. John Cairns writes in *Scientific American*, that **only about twenty or thirty people a year are being saved through chemotherapy for this disease.** For the common cancers, the **results have been more often negative than positive.** He also reminds us, many of the drugs used are known to be carcinogenic (cause cancers), and somewhere between 5 and 10 percent of the surviving patients get and die of leukemia, caused by the chemotherapy, in the first ten years after treatment.[16]

Many scientists have begun to question the basic premise of cancer chemotherapy, which is the use of toxic agents to kill every last cancer cell (virtually impossible) in the body. Dr. Victor Richards, for example, calls chemotherapy **"at best an**

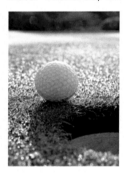

uncertain method of therapy" because it **cannot harm or kill cancer cells "without producing comparable effects on all normal cells."** In the limited situations where chemotherapy succeeds it is because it is a systemic poison, and it fails for the same reason. "With chemotherapy," Richards adds, "we have no sure shot…it is clear that **we can never eliminate the last cancer cell by using antimetabolites (chemotherapy)."**[17]

---

[16] Cairns, John. "The Treatment of Diseases and the War Against Cancer." *Scientific American* 253:51-9, November 1985.

[17] Richards, Dick. *The Topic of Cancer: When the Killing Has to Stop*. New York: Pergamon Press,1981.

PART I: Why Chemotherapy Does Not Work 97.9% of the Time[1]

It takes more than money to buy time.

CANCERS ANSWERS

EXCERPT FROM

VOLUME 1 ✦ PAGE 456
CANCERSANSWERS.ORG

the CANCER ESTABLISHMENT

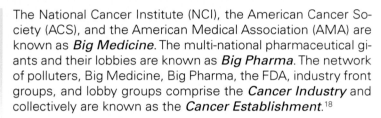

The National Cancer Institute (NCI), the American Cancer Society (ACS), and the American Medical Association (AMA) are known as *Big Medicine*. The multi-national pharmaceutical giants and their lobbies are known as *Big Pharma*. The network of polluters, Big Medicine, Big Pharma, the FDA, industry front groups, and lobby groups comprise the *Cancer Industry* and collectively are known as the *Cancer Establishment*.[18]

The main goal of these groups, according to *Cancer: Step Outside the Box* (2011), is to maintain the status quo and huge profits in the cancer industry.[19] Their techniques are simple and straightforward:

1. To suppress alternative cancer treatments and persecute/prosecute those who advocate alternative treatments, thereby eliminating competition that jeopardizes all the jobs and incomes in the industry.

2. To persuade (brainwash) the public to believe that chemotherapy (poisons), surgery (cutting/slashing/damaging), and radiation (burning/destroying) are the only three viable options for cancer treatment ("the Big 3"), thereby reducing and eliminating positive opportunities for cancer patients. And,

3. To aggressively promote and sell the Big 3, since the goal of the cancer industry is to survive and profit. Their survival takes precedence over yours. Their jobs actually turn out to be more important to them than our lives.

[18] Moss, Ralph W. *The Cancer Industry*. Pages 389-419. State College, PA, 1999, 2002.

[19] Bollinger, Ty. *Cancer: Step Outside the Box*. USA: Infinity 5102 Partners, 2011.

Your body is just another one for your doctor;
it's the only one for you.

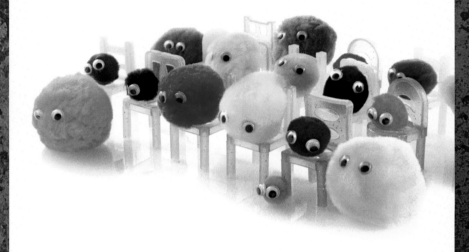

how IT ALL STARTED

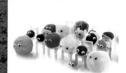

John D. Rockefeller decided in 1910 to expand his Standard Oil Company into chemicals and drugs by purchasing I.G. Farben, Europe's largest chemical and Drug Company. Second, he commissioned the Flexner Report which was submitted to the Carnegie Foundation, the gist of which said that our nation's medical schools were not teaching sound medicine, i.e., selling drugs and pharmaceuticals, and that a watchdog/gatekeeper was needed. The American Medical Association became that watchdog and was empowered to provide accreditation to all medical schools (required for funding).

Schools were required to drop courses like natural medicines, electro-medicine, homeopathy, and all other alternatives, or risk losing accreditation and funding. Half of all medical schools did lose their accreditation between 1910 and 1944. These monopolies have continued to this day. Rockefeller's domination plan continues to be a smashing success for the Big 3.[20, 21]

Anyone who disagreed with this approach was labeled and pursued as a quack. Studies that promoted biochemical or pharmaceutical approaches were funded; approaches that favored alternatives and nutrition were not funded and given a bad reputation and labeled as *snake oil*. For the most part, this outrageous conflict of interest of Big Pharma and Big Medicine continues with 100 years of momentum to this day. As candidly admitted by a recent NCI director, the NCI has **become a government pharmaceutical company**. However, Dr. Epstein chronicles in his book, *The Politics of Cancer Revisited*, how the cancer industry is suppressing mountains of evidence about environmental and other causes of cancer. [22]

[20] Ibid. Pages 4-7, 167.

[21] Moss, Ralph W. *The Cancer Industry*. Pages 391, 421. State College, PA, 1999, 2002.

[22] Epstein, Samuel S. *The Politics of Cancer*. San Francisco: Sierra Book Club, 1978.

A lifetime of believing a lie will not change the truth.

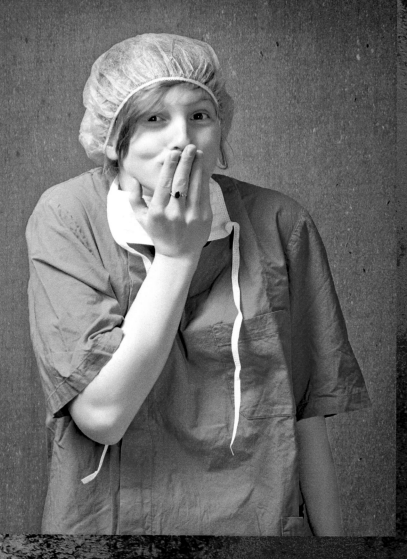

cancer IS AN INDUSTRY
PART III

Cancer is an industry providing billions of dollars annually to a wide variety of interests. Simple profit motive, personal self-interest, and politics each play a role in suppressing the truth about alternative treatments that can go well beyond surgery, chemotherapy and radiation. The huge profits available to the cancer industry provide all the financial incentive necessary to see alternative medicine suppressed. Simply stated, natural remedies are not as patentable and/or profitable as surgery, chemo and radiation, and are not enough for the medical profession to turn its interest from keeping their jobs and making high profits to new, less profitable treatments, even when they historically provide better results.

Annual cancer treatment costs can run easily from the $100,000's of dollars to about $850,000 per patient and up.[23] According to the National Institute of Health, about 12.5 million living Americans have cancer. According to the American Cancer Society, approximately 1.5 million people will be diagnosed with cancer this year for the first time, and almost 600,000 will die of the disease.[24] By 2020, annual expenditures for cancer treatment will reach between $157 billion and $207 billion, depending on the rate of inflation affecting cancer treatment costs, according to the Journal of the National Cancer Institute.[25]

[23] Moss, Ralph W. *Questioning Chemotherapy*. State College, PA: Equinox Press, October 8, 1996.
[24] American Cancer Society. A Twentieth Anniversary. In *Annual Report*. New York, 1965 *Cancer Facts and Figures*. New York, 1971, 1974, 1979, 1988 *Unproven Methods of Cancer Management*. New York, 1971, 1982, 1983,1986. Plants That Cure and Cause Cancer. *Cancer News 29*(2), Fall 1975.
[25] National Cancer Institute. *Fact Book*. DHEW Publication. Bethesda, MA, 1999. "Radiation Therapy for Cancer." Fact Sheet, 2010.

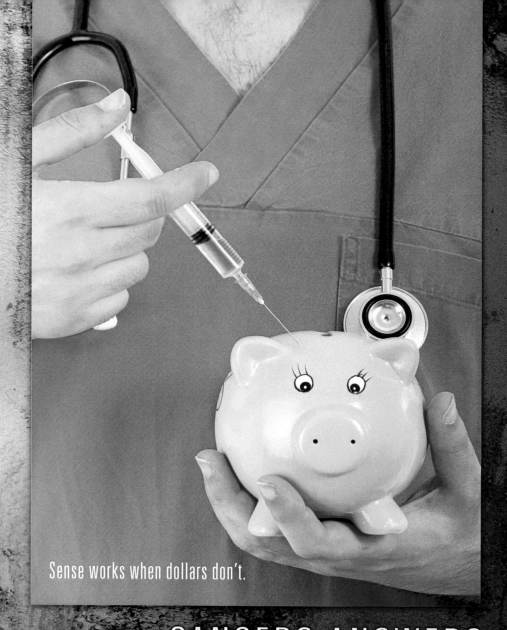

Sense works when dollars don't.

EXCERPT FROM CANCERS ANSWERS

VOLUME 1 ✦ PAGE 250

CANCERSANSWERS.ORG

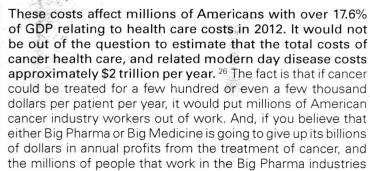

These costs affect millions of Americans with over 17.6% of GDP relating to health care costs in 2012. It would not be out of the question to estimate that the total costs of cancer health care, and related modern day disease costs approximately $2 trillion per year. [26] The fact is that if cancer could be treated for a few hundred or even a few thousand dollars per patient per year, it would put millions of American cancer industry workers out of work. And, if you believe that either Big Pharma or Big Medicine is going to give up its billions of dollars in annual profits from the treatment of cancer, and the millions of people that work in the Big Pharma industries will quit and walk away from their jobs, think again. It would be like the oil companies deciding to reduce the price of gasoline at the pump after charging this much for this long, or supporting and endorsing cheaper alternative energy sources – it's just not going to happen!

It's not in the cancer industry's financial interest to find an inexpensive *cure*, or *solution* for the cancer problem. The only parties with an incentive to find an alternative and inexpensive way to address cancer are the patients and families affected by this modern day *plague* themselves. The truth is that large numbers of cancer patients of all types are improving without conventional medicine by using alternative treatments every day. Even if doctors wanted to prescribe these alternative treatments after witnessing results from their own patients, they couldn't because the FDA does not approve them, or allow doctors to recommend anything not approved by the FDA. Because of the FDA's interaction and involvement with Big Pharma, the AMA, and a host of other private and government players, the FDA is largely controlled by political and financial considerations, not results.

[26] Wikipedia. http://en.wikipedia.org/wiki/Health_care_in_the_United_States

PART III: Cancer is an industry

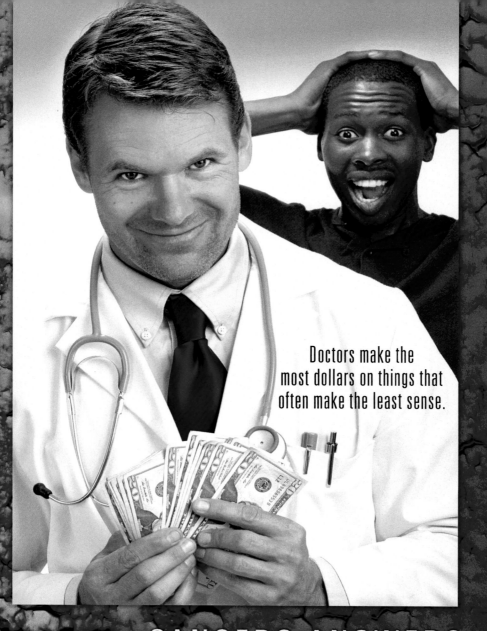

Doctors make the most dollars on things that often make the least sense.

understanding
CONVENTIONAL CANCER TREATMENT

Once there is a cancer diagnosis, the patient needs accurate treatment information and as many options as possible, and fast. We've often been brought up to believe that our doctors and physicians are our best source of dependable, accurate, trustworthy information, and that conventional treatments are the best and only options available. Certainly, most doctors believe that surgery, chemotherapy and radiation are the only answers to cancer treatment, as promoted by the cancer establishment. However, cancer is an industry, and like many businesses, is fraught with historic bias, traditional prejudice, conflicts of interest, and bureaucratic entanglements.

Surgery is more effective earlier in a diagnosis, although early enough is only relevant as to each individual case and usually an exercise in guesswork. In other words, cancer surgeons perform surgery, then hope that it was done *early enough,* which will only be determined over time. After the cancer and its *primary causes* have existed for long periods of time, have spread, or metastasized, which includes the majority of cancer cases, surgery can often do more damage and cause more problems than it solves. Additionally, the early stage of cancer is still extremely difficult to pin-point with conventional medical tests, and somewat risky, while medical mistakes rank as the 3rd leading cause of death in the U.S. Most researchers believe, and experience often proves, that surgery can initiate and promote metastasis and the spread of cancer.

Of course, the removal of entire organs and body parts is fraught with complications, not to mention, a basic lack of common sense and total loss of function(s) to the body. Additionally, surgery can never guarantee the complete removal of all cancer cells because it targets specific tumors and organs and does not address the conditions of other critical organs, the immune system, the entire body, all the cancer cells in other parts of the body, or any *primary causes*. And, you can't take back a surgery!

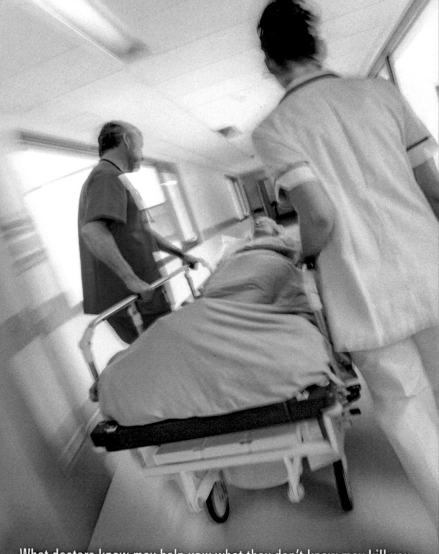

What doctors know may help you; what they don't know may kill you.

EXCERPT FROM CANCERS ANSWERS

VOLUME 1 ♦ PAGE 19

CANCERSANSWERS.ORG

For obvious economic reasons, chemotherapy is nearly always recommended after surgery in conventional cancer treatment. Even with the known risks and dangers to individuals (usually not known by the patient), it means lager profits for the doctors and Big Pharma that they are unwilling to leave on the table. Chemotherapy continues to be the norm in most cancer treatments despite the bad odds of it working at all, including the certain odds of increased future cancers and diseases, decreased quality of life, and shorter life-span.

Chemotherapy and radiation have far worse long-term recovery rates than surgery, and that's not saying much. **Because these treatments themselves are toxic** to cancer cells and healthy cells alike, the whole body is seriously compromised from that point on, making long-term recovery difficult at best, if not impossible. By severely damaging the immune system, as both chemo and radiation do, and filling the body with powerful toxic, poisonous agents, as chemo and radiation drugs do, many patients never recover from the treatment, let alone the cancer. **The patient gets the damage, the doctor gets the money, and the cancer gets the blame.**

Alternative, non-toxic treatments work by not harming the immune system, vital organs and the normal, healthy cells of the body. Conventional medicine typically practiced in the U.S. focuses on clubbing the cancer to death irrespective of the life, quality of life, and future of the patient. This approach is designed to primarily attack the tumors, which *never* represent all the cancer, or any of the *causes* in the body.

Alternative approaches focus on *treating the cance*r using the same method of *guessing* what the problem is (aka: diagnosis) and then *guessing* what to *try*. The main difference is that, generally they use less toxic substances to *try*. Doing less harm perhaps, but still *guessing*.

PART IV: Understanding Conventional Cancer Treatment

Guessing is no way
to accomplish a result.

EXCERPT FROM CANCERS ANSWERS

VOLUME 1 + PAGE 92
CANCERSANSWERS.ORG

Many cancer patients are never told that chemotherapy uses powerful chemicals that are carcinogenic (actually cause what they are being used to treat). These chemo agents often cause secondary cancers to develop in subsequent years, even if the patient initially survives. Radiation is well known to cause cancers. Chemo and radiation can also cause damage to our most critical organs such as the liver, kidneys, nerves, heart, and brain, and always damage our immune system which, in the end, is the main life force energy that truly protects, heals, and regenerates our body. These drugs can also severely damage and hamper the function(s) of the adrenals and thyroid glands, in addition to causing chronic pain and weakness throughout the body, effectively destroying, and further eliminating any quality of life. [27]

Once the immune system is compromised and special forces of the body are damaged, the cancer can continue to take over and spread even faster. **Cancer takes advantage of every low, slow, weak moment.** Now the damaged immune system is rendered incapable of fighting off the cancer, or even common infections, such as the common cold in many cases. It's difficult to understand how causing greater damage to the body will help the body recover long-term, yet that is the current thinking in the conventional treatment of cancer.

[27] Wikipedia. http://en.wikipedia.org/wiki/Chemotherapy.

PART IV: Understanding Conventional Cancer Treatment

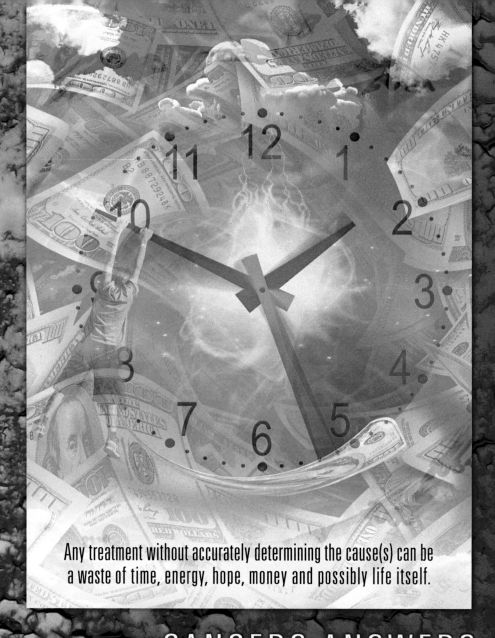

Any treatment without accurately determining the cause(s) can be a waste of time, energy, hope, money and possibly life itself.

EXCERPT FROM CANCERS ANSWERS

VOLUME 1 ✦ PAGE 50
CANCERSANSWERS.ORG

CANCER IS VIRTUALLY UNKNOWN IN
some cultures

In <u>Pharmacology Biochemistry & Behavior</u> (1984), Dr. Keith Brewer writes, "there are a number of areas where the incidences of cancer are very low. At the 1978 Stockholm Conference on Food and Cancer it was concluded that there is definitely a connection between the environment(s) and diet of these cultures and their low rate of cancer, but **since the relationship was not understood, no conclusions were drawn.**" [28]

The incidence of cancer among the Hopi Indians of Arizona is 1 in 1000 as compared to 1 in 2.5 for the USA as a whole. Fortunately, their food has been analyzed from the standpoint of nutritional values. In this study it was shown that the Hopi food runs higher than conventional foods in all the essential minerals. It is very high in potassium and exceptionally high in rubidium. Since their native soil is volcanic, it must also be very rich in cesium. These Indians live primarily on desert grown calico corn products. Instead of using baking soda they use the ash of chamisa leaves, a desert grown plant. The analyses of this ash showed it to be very rich in rubidium. The Indians also eat many fruits, especially apricots, per day. They always eat the kernels. They also have limited exposures in their natural environment.

Some 20 years ago the incidence of cancer among the Pueblo Indians of Arizona was the same as that for the Hopi Indians since their food was essentially the same. However, unlike the Hopi, these Indians have accrued certain items from outside their environment since supermarkets were installed in the area. Today the incidence of cancer among the Pueblos is 1 in 4, almost the same as the U.S.

[28] Bollinger, Ty. *Cancer: Step Outside the Box.* USA: Infinity 5102 Partners, 2011.

PART IV: Understanding Conventional Cancer Treatment

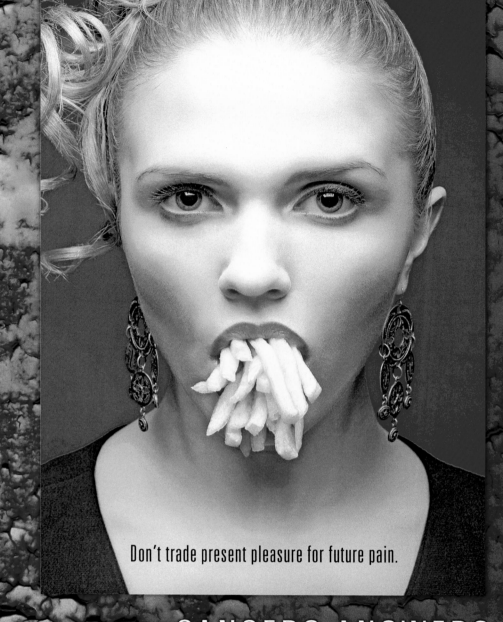

Don't trade present pleasure for future pain.

CANCER IS VIRTUALLY UNKNOWN IN
some cultures

It is reported that there is an increasing epidemic of cancer among this group. It must be emphasized here that the high incidence of cancer is likely not due to just what is in the supermarket foods, but additionally to what is not in it as well as the other changes in environment(s). It is essentially lacking natural minerals, anti-oxidants, rubidium and cesium and low in potassium and other minerals. They are continually increasing all the outside world exposures and contaminations we experience in metropolitan environments.

Cancer is essentially unknown among the Hunza of Northern Pakistan. They are, for the most part, vegetarians and are great fruit eaters. They drink at least 4 liters of natural mineral spring waters that abound in the area per day. This water has been analyzed and found to be very rich in minerals. Since the soil is volcanic in nature, it must be concluded that it will be rich in cesium and rubidium, as well as potassium.

The Indians who live in Central America and on the highland of Peru and Equador have very low incidences of cancer. The soil in these areas is volcanic. Fruit from the areas has been obtained and analyzed for rubidium and cesium and found to run very high in both elements and other minerals.

The Inuit of North America, the Aborigines and other hunter-gatherer groups have been studied for almost two hundred years. Suffice it to say that these groups did not and do not now eat a 100% raw food diet, as many believe. It can be noted that as far as plant foods go, at least, much of the cooking is done to neutralize native toxins in raw plants so that they can make use of what's available to them in their environment. They don't use particularly gentle methods of cooking either. And yet they have low cholesterol, and extremely low rates of heart disease and other degenerative diseases (Eaton 1996, 1985).

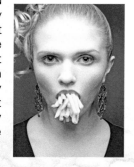

PART IV: Understanding Conventional Cancer Treatment

Your body is your business, and you need better management before you literally run your business into the ground.

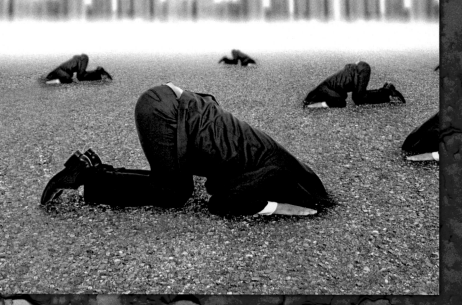

CANCER IS VIRTUALLY UNKNOWN IN
some cultures

It should be noted that hunter-gatherers experience many factors protective against cancer, such as: high antioxidant and fiber intake; virtually no exposure to pollution, chemicals, pesticides, or preservatives; and have a healthy vigorous lifestyle in general. Similarly, they enjoy many protective factors against cardiovascular disease (Eaton 1996, 1985). At least we can learn from the diet of hunter-gatherers that diseases of civilization were not born with the advent of fire. Hunter-gatherers have what appears to be a protective diet and invigorating lifestyle and much less exposure to the toxins, pathogens, and primary insults of metropolitan lifestyles.

A glance at *Eaton* (1996, 1985) shows that the incidence of diabetes and heart disease is extremely low, and their cholesterol levels are astonishingly low, ranging from roughly 105 to 145 in most cases (Eaton et al. 1988), especially given the high levels of cooked meat in their diet. They do suffer from some infectious diseases, and their lifespan is intermediate between that of developed nations and Third World agricultural nations. Which, given the lack of medical care, indicates the superiority of hunter-gatherers' diets and environments compared to basic rural, and agricultural environments and diets.

It is important to understand that while hunter-gatherers suffer from more infectious diseases than those of us living in modern sanitized conditions, so also do animals eating their native diet suffer from infectious diseases. **Diet is but one factor** in susceptibility to infectious disease.

The following is from *Food, Nutrition and the Prevention of Cancer: a Global Perspective,* World Cancer Research Fund (1997):

> It has often been said that cancer was rare among gatherer-hunter and pastoral peoples living in remote parts of the world, such as the Himalayas, the Arctic and equatorial Africa, when these peoples were first visited by explorers and missionaries (Williams 1908, Bulkley 1927, Schweitzer 1957). A summary of early accounts can be found in *Cancer Wars* (Proctor 1995).

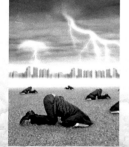

PART IV: Understanding Conventional Cancer Treatment

Being honest about a problem doesn't change it.

EXCERPT FROM CANCERS ANSWERS

VOLUME 1 ✦ PAGE 368

CANCERSANSWERS.ORG

CANCER IS VIRTUALLY UNKNOWN IN
some cultures

Such accounts have been taken to mean that cancer was generally rare in early history. The African explorer, Dr. David Livingstone, suggested that cancer is a "disease of civilization" (Maugh 1979). Practically nothing is known about rates of cancer until careful records were first kept in Europe in the eighteenth century. These suggest that, historically, cancer might have been a relatively uncommon disease, or just misdiagnosed as it is still today.[29]

Let's add that diet is not the only factor that can contribute to cancer. Recall that humans are exposed to many carcinogens (Ames 1990), and that smoking is quite common in hunter-gatherers (Bicchieri 1972). In addition, carcinogens themselves are not the only factors, or *causes* in the development of cancer, as many other aspects of environment(s) and lifestyles may play a significant role. For hunter-gatherer women, late onset of menarche (16 years old), having a first child at a relatively young age (19.5 on average), longer duration of breast-feeding (average length 2.9 years for each child), large average number of children (6), earlier menopause (47 years old), exercise throughout life, along with dietary habits all suggest the incidence of breast, uterus and ovary cancer were very low in comparison with rates seen among women in modern industrialized countries (Eaton 1994).[30]

We see similar disease-free results among the Hunzas, the Vilcabambans and the Georgian/Abkhasians. It's likely that their disease-reduced conditions result not so much from what is in their diets and environments, as what is *not* in their diets and environments. Note that when these groups adopt Western diets, their health deteriorates to Western levels suggesting that it is **not the role of genetics** at play in this equation. It appears that the nonexistence of common toxins, pathogens in their environment combined with traditional, nutrition rich, balanced diets prepared with their specific environmental foods contributes to their improved disease conditions.

---

[29] "Food, nutrition and the prevention of cancer: a global perspective," *World Cancer Research Fund* (1997).

[30] Bollinger, Ty. *Cancer: Step Outside the Box*. USA: Infinity 5102 Partners, 2011.

PART IV: Understanding Conventional Cancer Treatment

The biggest problems you can see
are often started by causes you can't.

CANCER IS A MODERN
lifestyle disease

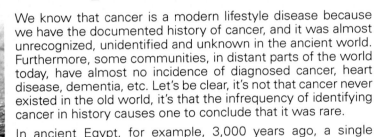

We know that cancer is a modern lifestyle disease because we have the documented history of cancer, and it was almost unrecognized, unidentified and unknown in the ancient world. Furthermore, some communities, in distant parts of the world today, have almost no incidence of diagnosed cancer, heart disease, dementia, etc. Let's be clear, it's not that cancer never existed in the old world, it's that the infrequency of identifying cancer in history causes one to conclude that it was rare.

In ancient Egypt, for example, 3,000 years ago, a single papyrus talks about a few cases of an illness that may have been cancer, but we can't be sure. More modern MRI testing of over 3,000 mummies found one single instance of cancer in all the mummies examined. According to the American Cancer society, half of all men and a third of all women today will develop diagnosable cancer in their lifetime.

In the Archives of Pathology and Laboratory Medicine (1991), Dr. Marc Micozzi recounts, "I tackled a huge project for the Walter Reed Army Medical Center and the National Cancer Institute (NCI). We researched every single case of cancer that had been recorded in prehistoric animals and ancient humans. And people were astounded by the results. There was no evidence of the common cancers that are found in the 20th and 21st centuries." [31]

The first *modern* cases of cancer show up in late 18th century England among chimney sweeps. Of course today, we all know not to inhale carcinogenic particles like engine exhaust and toxic chemicals that abound, but what about the hundreds of carcinogenic particles that we cannot smell or see, or microscopic live organisms that are in and on our food, water, and air? The first cases of surgical removal of cancer tumors are reported at that time by Scottish surgeon John Hunter and continue to this day.

[31] Micozzi, Marc S. *Insider's Cures.* Baltimore, MA: Insiders-Cures website. 2013.
Complementary and Integrative Medicine in Cancer Care and Prevention: Foundations and Evidence-Based Interventions. New York: Springer Publishing Company, 2006.
Fundamentals of Complementary and Alternative Medicine. New York: Saunders, 2010.

PART IV: Understanding Conventional Cancer Treatment

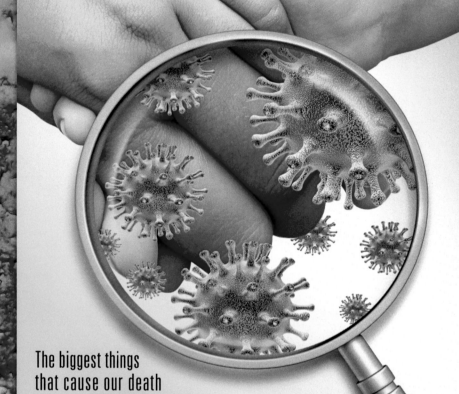

The biggest things
that cause our death
are the littlest things that
don't seem to bother us at all.

EXCERPT FROM CANCERS ANSWERS

VOLUME 1 + PAGE 408
CANCERSANSWERS.ORG

CANCER IS A MODERN
lifestyle disease

Cancer is a modern disease with real causes that increase with all our conveniences and improvements and exposures to our modern world and modern lifestyles. However, the modern approaches to managing cancer are more like *tortuous medieval* experiments. Including cutting (surgery), burning (radiation therapy), and poisoning (chemotherapy). These modern treatments are often worse on the patient than the disease.

Of course, the *hope* is that we kill the cancer before the patient dies from the treatment(s). But, in the majority of cases, while some tumors may shrink or be cut out, these treatments do n*othing* to extend and improve people's lives in the end. And in a big percent of cases, actually kill them sooner than the disease alone. All things considered, why wouldn't modern, *enlightened* medicine consider natural, safer alternatives? **The safety profile for natural medicine on average is over 20 times better than chemotherapy**, according to *Natural Compounds in Cancer Therapy* (2001). "What ever happened to the old medical oath: 'first do no harm?'" says Micozzi. [32]

The government does screen plants and natural products for anti-cancer activity, but they only look at substances with the ability to kill cancer cells by themselves. Agents that kill cancer cells are also toxic to normal cells. This is what causes the terrible side effects of chemotherapy. On the other hand, nature contains remarkable plant substances that have been discovered to work in multiple and beneficial ways throughout the body. Some can initiate cancer cell death without harming healthy cells, and can even transform cancer cells back toward normal cells under very specific circumstances. This is a process called re-differentiation. This is a remarkable fact of nature. And, it's completely ignored by the *cancer establishment*.

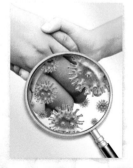

[32] Ibid.

You may be repeating the history you haven't studied.

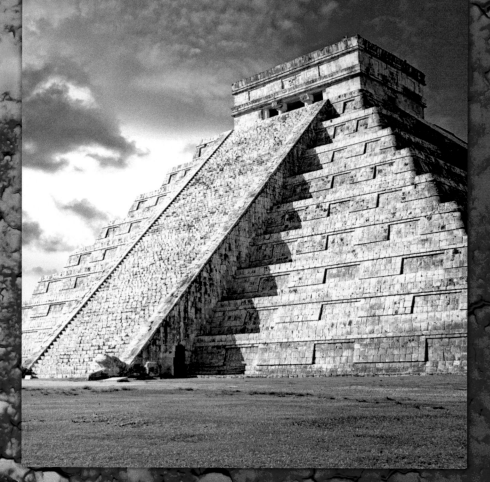

EXCERPT FROM CANCERS ANSWERS

VOLUME 1 ✦ PAGE 56
CANCERSANSWERS.ORG

lifestyle disease

"These plant substances have been known to Ayurvedic medicine (a form of healing native to India), and Chinese medicine for centuries. But, of course, most modern scientists remain proud of their ignorance of history and their view of its irrelevance to the marvelous medical achievements of the modern world. The secrets to fighting cancer are steeped in actual history," says Dr. Micozzi. [33]

Cancer was considered a *disease of modern civilization* due to its rapid increase since the turn of the 20th century. In Germany, it was declared the "number one enemy of the state" (1935). In fact, the Nazi war on cancer was the most aggressive in history. It included restrictions on the use of asbestos and bans on food dyes, pesticides, and tobacco, and they emphasized physical activity, natural medicines, and a diet rich in fresh fruits and green vegetables. All in the 1930s and 1940s.

At about the same time, the English found over a dozen foods that seem to be protective against cancer. Including beetroot, bread (whole meal), cabbage, carrots, cauliflower, onions, turnips, and watercress. They also proposed that there was a substance in green vegetables that was worth researching further. Keep in mind, the majority of vitamins had not yet been discovered in 1929 and

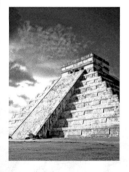

they did not completely understand why any of these tendencies occurred. Fifteen years later, they repeated the study focusing on green vegetables. Researchers found they provided some protection against lung, gastrointestinal, and other cancers. But, unfortunately for us, all this research fell on deaf ears and was swept under the rug. **You can't learn from the past if you outright ignore it. We must study history, or we're doomed to repeat it.**

[33] Ibid.

PART IV: Understanding Conventional Cancer Treatment

The only thing worse than having Cancer is not knowing why.

EXCERPT FROM CANCERS ANSWERS

VOLUME 1 ✦ PAGE 7

CANCERSANSWERS.ORG

lifestyle disease

The U.S. launched its own *War on Cancer* in 1972. The U.S. scientists and researchers started from scratch, ignoring years of research earlier in the century and all the wisdom of the Ancients. A second front opened in 1982 and The National Academy of Sciences Food and Nutrition Board issued a report on *Diet and Cancer*. This report summarized the potential of diet and nutrition in *promoting*, or *preventing* cancer. Medical science understood very little about human nutrition at the time. So much of the new *crash program research* had to be directed to studying basic aspects of how vitamins and nutrients are arranged in foods and how they enter the bloodstream and tissues of the human body instead of what benefits they provide to the body, or their cancer fighting abilities.

"The NIH and their advisors and lead scientists made many mistakes that have been documented. One was insisting that testing nutrients should be done only one at a time. Nutrients exist in nature as rich, complex combinations in natural, harmonic, resonant energetic balance in their fresh, live state. Even if they found some success, this approach would delay finding the *whole* truth and virtually guarantee the war on cancer would be delayed for at least another generation. All the while, chemotherapy doctors and their drug company profits would continue to stack up," says Micozzi. [34]

"The NCI slogged along *guessing* down the wrong roads for many years. Following this misdirected, *unnatural* approach, they shamefully lacked a genuine understanding of the human anatomy and its functions that promote health and utilize nutritional substances. These basic aspects of human diet and nutrition were grossly ignored, under-studied and under-funded, neglected, and discarded as unimportant. All because the money had gone to the *big guns* of cutting, burning, drugging, and poisoning (the main profits for doctors, their employees and the cancer industry), instead of more natural and safer approaches (less suffering and misery for patients)," said Micozzi.

[34] Ibid.

PART IV: Understanding Conventional Cancer Treatment

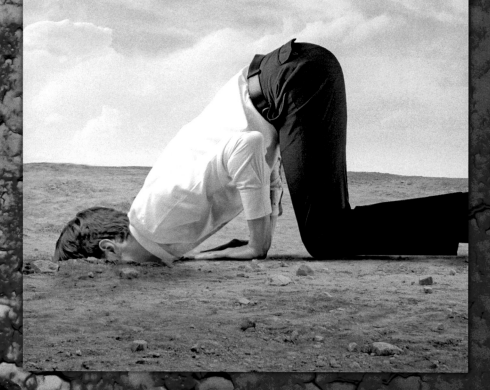

We live and die mostly by our ignorance.

EXCERPT FROM CANCERS ANSWERS

VOLUME 1 ✦ PAGE 14

CANCERSANSWERS.ORG

CANCER IS A MODERN
lifestyle disease

"Great strides were made in research at the time, all of which was promptly ignored by doctors and the cancer establishment. A report in 1984 tracking the epidemiological studies of 46 research studies showed that 33 of the studies showed that vitamin C offered significant protection against some cancers…particularly for esophageal, pancreatic, stomach, lung, and breast cancers. That's a 71% rate of positive results. These results were later reported in *Nutrition and Cancer Prevention: Investigating the Role of Micronutrients* (1989). It seems that the powers that be at NIH in 1984 had invested heavily in a substance that would later prove to be a failure in cancer research: beta-carotene, a plant derived form of Vitamin A. Years of wasted research and tens, even hundreds of millions of dollars later, this *then media darling* was found to be ineffective. Well, the *powers that be* were not to be *embarrassed* again, so serious studies into nutrition as preventative care, or treatment of cancer has been largely ignored to this day by the NIH and the CDC. The USDA and the Department of Energy continue to fund studies in this area, and do appear to be interested in the truth about some nutrition, but nothing at the levels required for the probable breakthroughs we need today in cancer research. The cancer authorities today would rather be ignorant, unreceptive, and resistant, than embarrassed (wrong)," says Dr. Micozzi.[35]

Today we know about a myriad of nutrients that promote good health and improve bodily functions. We also know about many factors, including alternative and complimentary protocols that improve the odds of dealing with cancer, and we know that it can and should be done with natural, non-toxic, empowering protocols, by average brave patients and their alternative professional guides (experienced in actual results beating cancer, not just treating cancer).

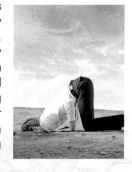

[35] Ibid.

PART IV: Understanding Conventional Cancer Treatment

When you make the body weaker, you make the Cancer stronger.

EXCERPT FROM CANCERS ANSWERS

VOLUME 1 + PAGE 95
CANCERSANSWERS.ORG

one size DOES NOT FIT ALL

It is vital to properly and professionally strengthen the immune system and other special forces of the body while effectively eliminating toxins and foreign invaders (pathogens, live organisms, microbes, toxins, etc.) in your battle against cancer and its primary causes. This is especially true if you are getting medical treatments like chemo and radiation (poisons) that slow down and damage your immune system and special forces of your body. Many natural supplements and alternative protocols (like electro-medicine instruments) *power up* energies of the cells, tissues, organs, and systems of the body and power up the immune system and all special forces of the human organism. This is why so many of them are touted as being able to help you improve your body's odds of beating cancer.

Unfortunately, **most cancer patients have more seriously compromised immune systems** that a supplement, or group of supplements, would not work well enough to perform effectively enough to win this battle. This compromised immune system with other normal bodily functions, like digestion, assimilation, elimination, and healing weakened and/or damaged, make it even more difficult to compete against this opponent. This is why it can be so difficult to decide what protocols to use because there are so many quality of life issues in the mix, in addition to having the overwhelming challenge of cancer. If a supplement, product, or protocol has been used for years, especially if it is popular, you'll hear how many people *think* it has beat a cancer. The **problem** is that you **don't know if it actually worked** 2% of the time, or 50% or more, and on **what conditions an individual's body was in at that time**; their unique combination of cause(s), types, quantity and grade of cancer; and differences in personal history, exposures, environments and lifestyles. Given the number of people who die from cancer, the success rate of most supplements and protocols is fairly low. It is easy to squander money and, more importantly, time, energy, and hope on products and protocols that won't make enough of a difference to accomplish a *noticeable* result. Clearly, an *experienced guide* is necessary to assist the cancer patient in this *guessing* process. The problem is never too much, or too many protocols, but rather the right *effective* treatments, fast enough, to slow the cancer down, determine and eliminate the primary cause(s), and turn the condition(s) of that individual body around.

PART IV: Understanding Conventional Cancer Treatment

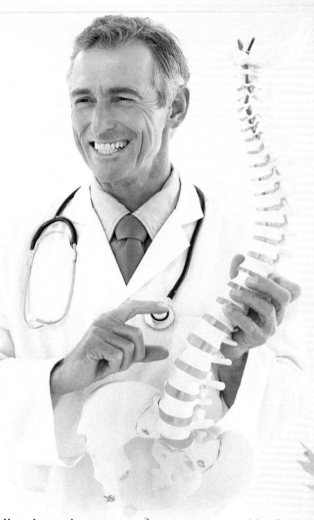

Is it really what a doctor says that means something?
Or, does he just believe you can't figure it out?

EXCERPT FROM CANCERS ANSWERS

VOLUME 1 ✦ PAGE 136
CANCERSANSWERS.ORG

one size DOES NOT FIT ALL

The causes of each and every cancer situation vary while our individual immune systems are each different and under the influence of different histories, experiences, stresses and exposures. Effective treatments must be focused on the specific individual patient and his/her unique conditions and combination of causes. Cancer is much more difficult to control when the individual is in a very weakened physical conditions. Their kidneys, adrenals, liver, intestines, and other critical organs involved in the functions of the immune system will lack the energy to be able to handle the large number of pathogens, toxins, microbes, poisons, and microscopic organisms and toxic wastes stored up in the body. Importantly, all of these and other contaminants must be eliminated to win the battle against causes, weaknesses, infections, and the resulting cancer itself. Individualized products and protocols that actually strengthen, power up, energize, and support improved functions of the body so that it becomes strong enough to effectively mount a battle to eliminate the cancer must be found and analyzed. Often times the body must be detoxified and strengthened before certain protocols can be tolerated, or be the most effective.

By only *guessing* and *trying* suggested products and protocols, cancer patients get fatigued and drained of the life-force energy they need to compete. Their body has been working hard 24/7 managing and fighting ALL the causes (often unknown by the patient or doctors) for all the years the patient has had them, without even being aware of the causes, or doing anything about eliminating them until realizing the body is now *shutting down*. When the body is weak enough, long enough, and lacks the strength and energy to handle the causes and the resulting symptoms (cancer), then surgery, chemotherapy, radiation, and other experimental drugs are even more likely to be the straw that breaks the camel's back.

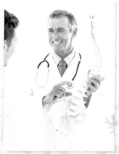

PART IV: Understanding Conventional Cancer Treatment

Positive results are more skills than pills.

help

one size DOES NOT FIT ALL

Having cancer is *like being lost in a jungle*. You are not going to guess your way out of the inherent dangers of being lost in a foreign, perilous, uncharted territory, like the cancer world. You might think all you would need is survival gear or supplies. While those things might help and/or be useful in order to *make it* and actually live through the ordeal, you mostly need *guidance* for the right direction and navigation all the way out of danger. The cancer patient needs someone who knows all the dangers to be avoided and the effective methods to be used under all the different circumstances that can arise. It would be like being lost and having a native guide, or warrior, appear with actual experience in "rescuing others" and real previous experience dealing with the vast array of emergency situations that can and do arise on this journey.

The only way to be certain about which dietary changes, appropriate supplements and protocols to use is to find the services of the *most* objective, experienced and competent alternative practitioners and consultants available and continue to search for those with the most objective, actual experience. Please remember that there's more to actually *beating* cancer than changing, or improving one's diet (eating more veggies, taking extra vitamins, supplements), or saying one *believes* in something. The most successful treatments are always thoughtful, individualized, complex, aggressive, accurately recommended, and don't waste a lot of time. This type of guidance is rare and may save your life. Choose thoughtfully and wisely.

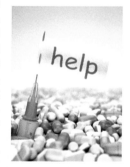

PART IV: Understanding Conventional Cancer Treatment

Fitting in will take you out.

EXCERPT FROM CANCERS ANSWERS

VOLUME 1 + PAGE 260
CANCERSANSWERS.ORG

the immune SYSTEM

We are all born with pre-cancerous cells. How long do we need to be on this planet; how many places do we have to go; or how many exposures (unseen, unknown, and unnoticed by any body) do we need to have in this world until these irritated, inflamed, acidic, poisoned, cells get weakened and damaged enough to replicate as damaged foreign looking cells? Cancerous cells (weak, damaged, abnormal) are always being created in the body as a result of irritating, inflaming, injuring, damaging, exposure(s) inside the body. It's an ongoing process that has gone on since your birth.

Cancer has exploded in the second half of the twentieth century due in part to the excessive and ever-increasing amounts of toxins, pathogens, microscopic organisms, and pollutants we are all exposed to continually. Combine high stress lifestyles that drain energy, minerals, oxygen, and strength from the body, with a weakened immune system and overworked special forces of the body, and you have a formula for the disaster, we call cancer. The problems continue to mount with a common lack of proper nutrition. Cancer is actually the "ultimate chronic infection," and all infections begin with deficiencies, causes, and the increase in number of chemical additives to our entire food supply (approximately 20,000 new chemicals are introduced every year!). We are living with the continual increase in exposures to pathogens; poor quality junk food that's full of pesticides, chemicals, bacteria, microscopic organisms that are irradiated and now genetically modified; as well as environmental exposures -- such as electromagnetic stress (EMFs), artificial light, and just about everything else that wasn't here 200 years ago. It turns out that Cancer is not just a manmade *modern lifestyle* disease, it's a disease of ignorance and denial, and it is **CAUSED**.

PART IV: Understanding Conventional Cancer Treatment

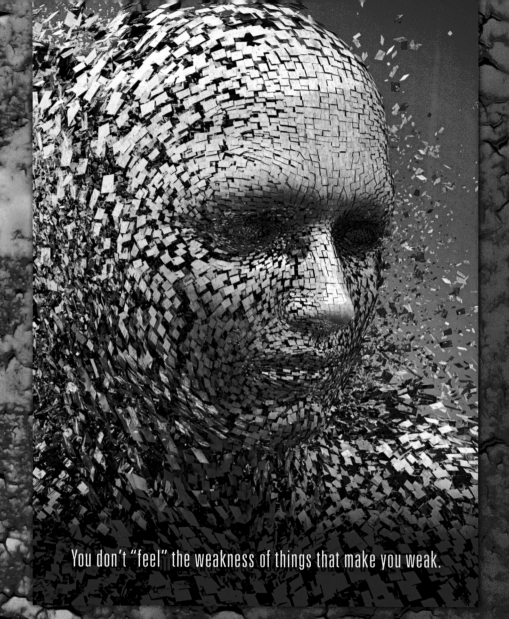

You don't "feel" the weakness of things that make you weak.

EXCERPT FROM CANCERS ANSWERS

VOLUME 1 + PAGE 396
CANCERSANSWERS.ORG

the immune SYSTEM

All these common life exposures are *assaults* on the body that weaken the immune system and change the internal environment in the body to an environment that permits and produces the presence and spread of cancer. The body gets conditioned and weakened to the point that it will tolerate the presence of cancer, and promote the growth and spread of cancer allowing causes to continue to breed and feed more cancer(s). Cancer is not a mysterious disease that suddenly attacks you out of the blue. *Cancer is not a disease you treat, it's an enemy you must beat.* It has primary causes and contributing factors that you MUST identify and eliminate when you can access the knowledge, experience, skills, and tools necessary.

Cancer tumors begin when more cancerous cells are being created than a weakened, overworked, depleted immune system can control and eliminate. Constant exposure to tens of thousands of manmade chemicals from birth onward, chlorinated and fluoridated water, electromagnetic pollution (man-made negative energies), pesticides, chemicals and other toxins, lead to the creation of too many free radicals and excessive numbers of damaged cells. This alone would be enough to increase cancer levels when combined with an immune system weakened by a life-long diet of dead, over-cooked, refined and over-processed, contaminated foods.

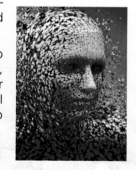

At some point, the body is no longer able to keep weaknesses, deficiencies, infections, pathogens, and the resulting cancer under control. As this continues, cancer will continue to express, manifest and show up in multiple parts of the body.

PART IV: Understanding Conventional Cancer Treatment

Doing nothing is one of the Primary Causes of Cancer.

EXCERPT FROM CANCERS ANSWERS

VOLUME 1 ✦ PAGE 37
CANCERSANSWERS.ORG

the immune SYSTEM

Overcoming cancer is a process of reversing the conditions and causes that influenced the body to produce the cancer. Knowing the exact primary causes is the greatest help to correct those conditions, as it is with solving any other problem in this *cause* and *affect* world. What you need to do is to strongly, dramatically, and quickly interrupt and reverse the cancer-causing conditions in the body and and professionally modify lifestyle so that the body becomes stronger, healthier, provides more power to the immune system, and stops breeding, feeding and strengthening the cancer and its causes. The more cancer there is, the more serious the physical condition(s), indicating that much more has to be done, done effectively, and done faster. We need to learn from mistakes. There are two kinds of mistakes we are obligated to learn from in this life: our own, and, the mistakes of others -- the latter is the preferred!

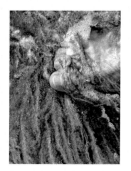

Try rhymes with *die*. There is not enough time to *re-make* all the mistakes all those other cancer patients before us have made. After all, they all died guessing and trying. *Don't let personal likes & dislikes interfere with potential!*

When it comes to vehicles, like your body, how well they're maintained is how well and how long they operate.

EXCERPT FROM

CANCERS ANSWERS

VOLUME 1 + PAGE 194

CANCERSANSWERS.ORG

There are Worse Things than Cancer: Conventional
cancer treatment

Chemotherapy is toxic, carcinogenic, destroys red blood cells, devastates the immune system, and destroys vital organs while weakening and damaging functions of the body. Chemotherapy wrecks the body so badly that it causes your hair to fall out, you are constantly nauseated, sick, and vomit uncontrollably. You are frequently dizzy with severe headaches and your immune system is permanently damaged, while cells and tissues are destroyed. Once upon a time, drugs derived from World War I, like nitrogen mustard gas experiments, showed destruction of fast growing tissues. Because cancer is made up of fast growing cells, the leap was made that these poisons might kill cancer cells. And they were right. Chemotherapy kills cancer cells and shrinks tumors. It also indiscriminately kills healthy cells, damages and weakens cells, tissues, vital organs and systems of the body, while weakening and interfering with all normal functions of the human organism. In fact, **early tests of chemotherapy on leukemia killed 42% of all patients** that were treated with it (When Healing Becomes a Crime, by Ausubel).[37] At their autopsies, the cancer tumors had shrunk, but they were dead! What we now know from Dr. Ralph Moss in his book *Questioning Chemotherapy*, is that **the shrinking of tumors has no effect on long term longevity and cancer survival rates**. *(Ibid.)*

According to Clinical Oncology (December 2004), the *actual 5-year survival rate of American adults using chemotherapy is 2.1%*, or slightly less than the 5-year survival rate of adults who receive no treatment at all for their cancer.[38] Dr. Alan Levin M.D. in his book **Dissent in Medicine - 9 Doctors Speak Out**, says categorically that **"most cancer patients in this country die of chemotherapy, not cancer."** Chemotherapy does not eliminate breast, colon, or lung cancer, which three count for the vast majority of cancers. This fact has been documented for over a decade, yet doctors still insist on chemotherapy for these tumors.

---

[37] Ausubel, K. *When Healing Becomes a Crime: The Amazing Story of the Hoxsey Cancer Clinics and the Return of Alternative Therapies.* Healing Arts Press, Rochester, NY, 2000.

[38] Morgan, G., Ward, R., and Barton, M. PubMed.gov. from *Clinical Oncology (R Coll Radioll)* 2004, Dec; 16(8):549-60.

PART IV: Understanding Conventional Cancer Treatment

It takes good scientists
to come up with bad science.

cancer treatment

In his book, *The Topic of Cancer: When the Killing Has to Stop*, Dick Richards cites a number of autopsy studies that have shown that cancer patients died from conventional treatments before the tumor had a chance to kill them. Dr. Ralph Moss writes convincingly "the amount of toxic chemicals needed to kill every last cancer cell was found to kill the patient long before it eliminated the tumor."

Most people are shocked to learn that chemotherapy causes cancer, but this is an undeniable fact. A study done at the McGill Cancer Center in Montreal surveyed sixty-four oncologists to see how they personally would respond to a cancer diagnosis. Fifty-eight of the sixty-four oncologists (90.6%) said that chemotherapy was unacceptable for them and their family members due to the fact that the drugs don't work and are toxic to everyone's system (*Cancer: Why We're Still Dying to Know the Truth* by Philip Day).

"Cancer is a disease which always results from a compromised immune system. Chemotherapy is known to devastate the immune system," writes Ty Bollinger in his book Cancer: Step Outside the Box. "How can you cure a disease which results from a compromised immune system with a drug which further compromises and even damages and destroys the immune system?"

In 1991, German epidemiologist Dr. Ulrich Abel published a comprehensive analysis of every major study and clinical trial of chemotherapy that had ever been done in The Lancet (August 1991). "Success of most chemotherapies is appalling...There is no scientific evidence for its ability to extend in any appreciable way the lives of patients suffering from the most common organic cancers...Chemotherapy for malignancies too advanced for surgery, which accounts for 80% of all cancers, is a scientific wasteland." At that time, Dr. Abel may have known more about chemotherapy than anyone else on Earth, yet his comprehensive study was buried and never again saw the light of day.

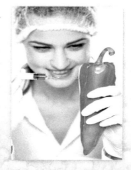

PART IV: Understanding Conventional Cancer Treatment

It's not what remission means to you,
it's what it means to Cancer: PERMISSION.

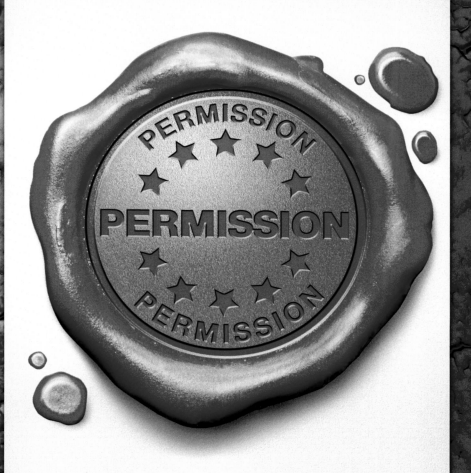

EXCERPT FROM CANCERS ANSWERS

VOLUME 1 + PAGE 16

CANCERSANSWERS.ORG

cancer treatment

Dr. Glenn Warner, a cancer specialist of note said: "We have a multi-billion dollar industry that is killing people, right and left, just for financial gain. Their idea of research is to see whether two doses of this poison is better than three doses of that poison."

Dr. Alan Nixon, past president of the American Chemical Society asserts, "As a chemist trained to interpret data, it is incomprehensible to me that physicians can ignore the clear evidence that chemotherapy does much, much more harm than any possible good."

French cancer specialist Dr. Charles Mathe says, "If I contracted cancer, I would never go to a standard cancer treatment Centre. Only cancer victims who live far from such cancer centers have a chance."

Dr. Dean Burk wrote a letter to his boss at the NCI condemning the institute's policy of continuing to endorse chemotherapy drugs when **everyone knew that they didn't work and caused cancer**. He argued: "Ironically, virtually all of the chemotherapeutic anti-cancer agents now approved by the Food and Drug Administration (FDA) for use in human cancer patients are (1) highly, or variously toxic at applied dosages; (2) markedly immuno-suppressive, that is, destructive of the patient's native resistance to a variety of diseases and causes, including the cancer; and (3) usually highly carcinogenic (makes that cancer worse and causes more cancers)... These now well established facts have been reported in numerous publications from the National Cancer Institute itself, as well as throughout the United States, and, indeed, the world." Strangely, scientists at Sloan Kettering interpreted these same results as successful, because cancer tumors had shrunk, even when the patients died from these treatments.

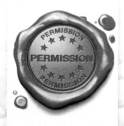

In the words of Mike Adams, **"Treating cancer with chemotherapy is like treating alcoholism with Vodka, or treating diabetes with high-fructose corn syrup. Cancer cannot be stopped by the very thing that starts it."**

PART IV: Understanding Conventional Cancer Treatment

If you think you know what to do,
how do you know when you're done?

EXCERPT FROM CANCERS ANSWERS

VOLUME 1 + PAGE 123

CANCERSANSWERS.ORG

Surgery

According to Dr. Patrick McGrady, **virtually all cancer surgery is unnecessary**. "Even though it's been proven conclusively that lymph node excision after radiation does not prevent the spread of cervical cancer, you will still see lymphadenectomies (lymph removal) performed all over the country routinely, **despite the fact that lymphadenectomies make women feel so bad they wish they were dead, and are a proven useless procedure**" (<u>Townsend Letter</u> June 1984).

According to Dr. Donald Kelley in his book, *One Answer to Cancer* he states, **"Often while making a biopsy the malignant tumor is cut, which tends to spread and accelerate the growth. Needle biopsies can accomplish the same tragic results."** A minute miscue or careless handling of tumor tissue by the surgeon or staff can literally spill millions of cancer cells into the cancer patient's bloodstream. Primary cancer (before metastasis) has about a 10 - 15% success rate using surgery. However, over 80% of cancer diagnoses occur after the primary cancer stage (recurrence), meaning **statistically the overall success rate of surgery in cancer treatment is less than 3%, a figure considerably higher than the success rate of chemotherapy and radiation**. Therefore, of the Big 3 conventional cancer treatments, surgery is by far the most effective (by a fraction of a percent). This provides **insight into how pathetic conventional cancer treatments actually are**.

One of the biggest problems with surgery, chemotherapy and radiation is that they are focused on treating the symptoms of cancer, i.e., the tumor(s), and not the causes of the cancer. Even though surgeons can sometimes remove a tumor, and chemotherapy and radiation can sometimes shrink the tumor, neither has any bearing on actually stopping the cancer, any of its causes, or extending the lifespan of the individual. The fact is that **tumor size has nothing to do with curing cancer** despite the oncological **obsession with tumor size** (the only thing they can see or show you). The tumor is the tip of the iceberg, the tail of the dragon, the dead leaf on the limb of your tree, the rattle on the rattlesnake, the flashing spot (first sign) that signals something has gone very wrong inside the body. **Without effectively identifying and eliminating the underlying *actual causes*, however, no cure is possible**.

PART IV: Understanding Conventional Cancer Treatment

"Being good" is a principle ingredient in losing any contest.

Radiation

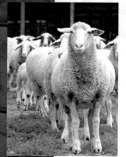

According to Dr. Lucian Israel in his well-known book, *Conquering Cancer* (1979), "Patients who undergo radiation therapy are more likely to have their cancer "metastasize" to other sites in their bodies. The radioactivity used to kill cancer cells also triggers the process of "DNA mutation" that creates new cancer cells of other types (more resistant and aggressive)."

The New England Journal of Medicine echoes these remarks in their September 1989 issue, "Secondary cancers are well known consistent complications of chemotherapy and radiation used to treat primary cancers."

In his book *Understanding Cancer*, John Laszlo (a former VP of Research at ACS) indicates that **when chemotherapy and radiation are used together, secondary tumors are 25 times more likely to occur than the normal rate.** Dr. Robert Jones writes in the Seattle Times (July 1980) that "**...many radiation complications do not occur until several years after treatment**, giving the practitioner and the patient a false sense of security for a year or two following therapy. The bone marrow, in which blood vessels are made, is largely obliterated in the field of irradiation...**This is an irreversible effect.**"

Dr. Jones continues, "Complications following high-dose radiation therapy for breast cancer are fibrous, shrunken breasts, rib fractures, pleural and/or lung scarring, nerve damage, scarring around the heart...suppression of all blood cells, and immune suppression." Now, cancer alone sounds pretty good compared to these multiple, automatic, guaranteed side effects.

The facts strongly suggest that treating cancer with radiation, a known carcinogen since X-rays were discovered in 1895, kills some cancer cells and **converts healthy cells to cancerous cells automatically and easily.** We've known for decades about the carcinogenic effect of radiation as it relates to X-rays in medicine and dentistry. Published reports indicate that over 80% of the first X-ray technicians and nurses developed cancer following their careers in medicine.

RADIATION:
NO SAFE AMOUNT!
ACCELERATES DEATH!

EXCERPT FROM CANCERS ANSWERS

VOLUME 1 + PAGE 430
CANCERSANSWERS.ORG

Radiation

According to the Archives of Internal Medicine (2009), CT scans cause at least 29,000 cases of cancer each year, and over 14,500 deaths annually in the U.S. alone. All because your doctor and you want to see the size of your tumor. Researchers found that patients are exposed to four times more radiation as estimated by earlier studies, equating one CT scan to the equivalent of 74 mammograms, or 442 chest X-rays! When radiation was developed, it was defined as: "NO SAFE AMOUNT!"...AND, "ACCELLERATES DEATH!" (It literally accelerates any, and all death processes (causes) in the human body...And, there are NO human senses that can perceive radiation. You cannot possibly know, or feel when you're exposed to any amount of radiation, as there are no human senses to make us aware of receiving any quantity at any time.

Pursuant to National Cancer Institute guidelines, there are many different types of targeted internal and external radiation therapies used in cancer treatment today. These vary, given differences in the type, size, location, tissue, distance the radiation needs to travel, etc. for the particular cancer. Plus, additional factors involving the patient's overall health, age, additional cancer therapies being used, and medical history must be considered. Combination therapies, i.e., radio-chemotherapy or chemo-radiation may kill more cancer cells, but will also cause additional negative side effects, long-term damage, and increases in other diseases while making real original primary causes worse.

According to the National Cancer Institute (NCI), **radiation therapy can cause both early (acute) and late (chronic) side effects**. Acute side effects occur during treatment, and chronic side effects occur months or even years after treatment ends. The side effects that develop depend on the area of the body being treated, the dose given per day, the total doses given, the patient's general medical and health condition, and other treatments given at the same time. Acute radiation side effects are caused by damage to rapidly dividing normal cells in the area being treated. These effects include skin irritation or damage at regions exposed to the radiation beams, and permanent weakening and damage to any healthy cells exposed. Examples include damage to the salivary glands or hair loss when the head or neck area is treated, or urinary problems when the lower

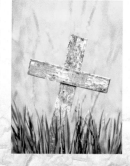

PART IV: Understanding Conventional Cancer Treatment

RADIATION:
The only thing that will rise
from those ashes is more fire.

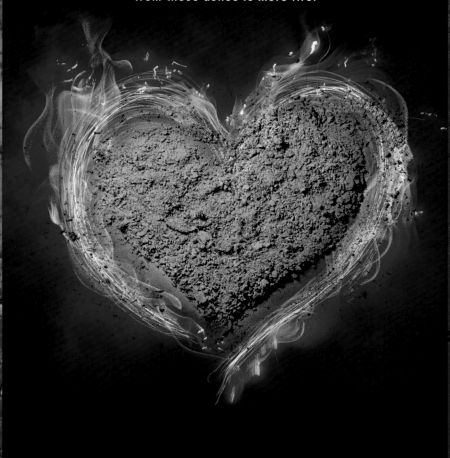

EXCERPT FROM CANCERS ANSWERS

VOLUME 1 + PAGE 405
CANCERSANSWERS.ORG

Radiation

Most acute noticeable effects disappear after treatment ends, though some can be permanent, like salivary gland damage, other healthy cells, tissues, organs, and systems of the body. Chronic fatigue is a common side effect of radiation therapy regardless of which specific part of the body is treated. Nausea, with, or without vomiting, is common! Chronic fatigue is treated and occurs sometimes when another part of the body like the brain is treated. Medications are available to help prevent or treat nausea and vomiting during treatment, but the damage is still done.

Latent side effects of radiation therapy may also occur. Depending on the area of the body treated, later side effects can include fibrosis (the replacement of normal tissue with scar tissue, leading to restricted movement of the affected area and other limitations), damage to the bowels (a big part of the immune system) causing diarrhea and bleeding, memory loss, infertility, and secondary cancers caused by any radiation exposure.

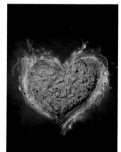

Secondary cancers may develop after radiation therapy no matter what part of the body is treated. For example, girls treated with radiation to the chest for Hodgkin's Lymphoma have an increased risk of developing breast cancer later in life. In general, the lifetime risk of a second cancer is highest in younger people treated for cancer as it has more time to deteriorate, degenerate, and weaken the body.

We need to see things how they are,
not just how they appear.

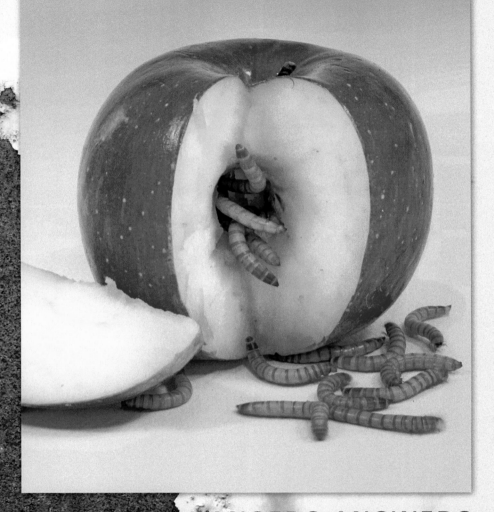

EXCERPT FROM CANCERS ANSWERS

VOLUME 1 + PAGE 501
CANCERSANSWERS.ORG

HOW CONVENTIONAL TREATMENTS HAVE failed

Why chemotherapy doesn't work –
Cancer tumors confirmed to have stem cells that regenerate tumors.

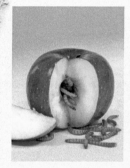

From a recent article by Jonathan Benson of *Natural News*, three recent studies published in the journals *Nature and Science* shed new light on why chemotherapy, a common conventional treatment for cancer, is typically a complete failure at permanently eradicating cancer. Based on numerous assessments of how cancer cells multiply and spread, researchers from numerous countries have confirmed that cancer tumors generate their own *stem cells*, which in turn breed and feed the continued growth and re-growth of new tumors after earlier ones have been removed, or eliminated.[39]

In one of the studies published in the journal *Nature*, researcher Luis Parada from the University of Texas (UT) Southwestern Medical Center in Dallas and his colleagues decided to investigate how new tumors are able to re-grow after previous ones have been removed with surgery and apparently wiped out with chemotherapy. To do this, Parada and his team identified and genetically labeled cancer cells in brain tumors of mice before proceeding to treat the tumors with conventional procedures and chemotherapy.

What they discovered was that, although chemotherapy appeared in some cases to reduce the size of the tumor and temporarily appeared to slow the growth and spread of some of the cancer, the treatment ultimately failed to stop new tumors from forming, or spreading. And the culprit, it turns out, was cancer stem cells that remained and persisted after the surgery and chemotherapy, which unsuspectingly stimulated the re-growth of new tumors at the same site and other locations in the body.

---

[39] Benson, Jonathan. "Why chemotherapy doesn't work – Cancer tumors confirmed to have stem cells that regenerate tumors." *Natural News.com*, 2012.

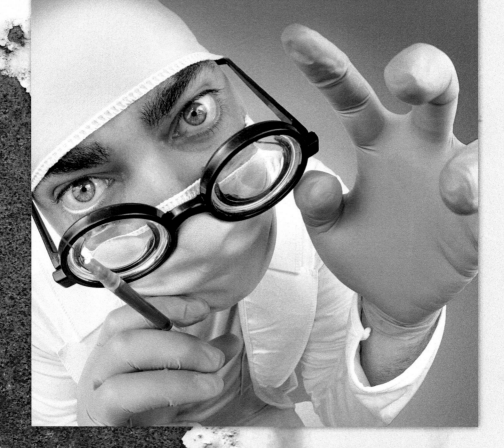

Most treatments for symptoms or diagnoses make most "real causes" worse.

EXCERPT FROM CANCERS ANSWERS

VOLUME 1 + PAGE 417
CANCERSANSWERS.ORG

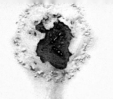

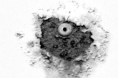

failed

Why chemotherapy doesn't work –
Cancer tumors confirmed to have stem cells that regenerate tumors.

A second study published in *Nature* found similar results using skin tumors, while a third published in the journal *Science* confirmed both of the other studies in research involving intestinal polyps. It appears as though, all across the board, cancer tumors possess an inherent ability to produce their own stem cells which can freely circulate throughout the entire body and develop into tumors. Traditional cancer treatments do absolutely *nothing* to affect these generators of new cancer cells.

Researchers at the *University of Michigan's* (UM) Comprehensive Cancer Center seem to agree with these conclusions as well, and are now suggesting, along with many others, a completely new approach to cancer treatment. "Rather than continue to rely on chemotherapy, radiation, and surgery, which we here at *Natural News* have long been warning our readers that they are all totally ineffective, progressive cancer researchers believe it is now time to move forward with investigating new treatment approaches." [40]

"Traditional cancer therapies like surgery, chemotherapy, and radiation **do not destroy the small number of cells driving the cancer's growth**," according to a statement released by UM's Comprehensive Cancer Center.

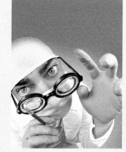

"Instead of trying to kill all the cells in a tumor with chemotherapy or radiation, we believe it would be more effective to use treatments targeted directly at these so-called cancer stem cells and identify other primary causes in the body. If the stem cells were eliminated, or what caused them, then the cancer would be unable to grow and spread to other locations in the body." [41]

---

[40] Ibid.
[41] Ibid.

PART V: How Conventional Treatments Have Failed

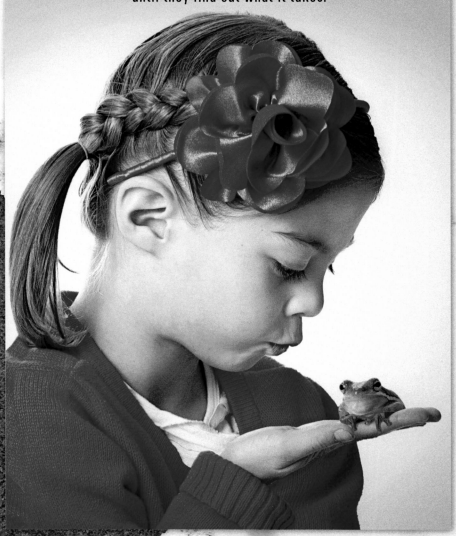

Most people are willing to do whatever it takes,
until they find out what it takes.

EXCERPT FROM

CANCERS ANSWERS

VOLUME 1 ♦ PAGE 66

CANCERSANSWERS.ORG

defining
THE STATISTICS
AND CONVENTIONAL STRATEGIES

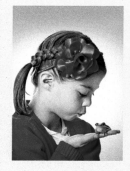

Organized medicine devoted to cancer research, treatment and education is led primarily by The American Cancer Society (ACS), the Food and Drug Administration (FDA), the National Cancer Institute (NCI), the American Medical Association (AMA), major pharmaceutical companies and cancer centers throughout the country. While these institutions claim cure rates of 40 - 50%, the reality is that their **methodology used to create these statistics is seriously flawed** in order to present a substantially better picture of their "cure rate." The reality is that once the veil is lifted (facts are revealed), the actual cure rate is closer to 2 - 3% of all cancer patients, according to most cancer researchers not in the cancer establishment, and outside the cancer industry.

Primary cancer, that cancer located early enough for surgical removal prior to metastasis, **has about a 15% cure rate**, possibly a little less. However, **the long-term survival rate of cancer patients using conventional treatment is about 1% or less** where the cancer has metastasized[42], according to most researchers, including Ralph Moss, author of numerous books including *The Cancer Industry, Questioning Chemotherapy, and Cancer Therapy: The Independent Consumer's Guide to Non-Toxic Treatment and Prevention.*

[42] Morgan, G., Ward, R., and Barton, M. PubMed.gov. from Clinical Oncology (R Coll Radioll) 2004, Dec; 16(8):549-60.

PART V: How Conventional Treatments Have Failed

You miss one turn on a map to the gold...
no gold for you!

EXCERPT FROM CANCERS ANSWERS

VOLUME 1 + PAGE 164
CANCERSANSWERS.ORG

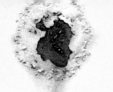

defining
THE STATISTICS
AND CONVENTIONAL STRATEGIES

There are numerous ways they have *manipulated* the statistical, conventional, medical cancer treatment success rates:[43]

1. **How *Cure* is Defined** – Just alive for five (5) years after diagnosis does not mean cancer free, or even good health.[44]

2. **Relative Survival Rate** - The Relative Survival Rate discounts/reduces the number of cancer deaths by adjusting for patients who may have died by other means, e.g., being run over by a bus.[45]

3. **Deletion of Patients Who Die Before Treatment is Completed** - If the patient dies of cancer before the cancer treatment protocol is completed, he/she is dropped from the cancer death rate statistics (in school they call this cheating).[46]

4. **Inserting statistics of non life-threatening cancer types** - Simple cancers like skin cancers that are easily treated are added to more serious cancer cure rates.[47]

5. **Exclusion of Certain Groups** - Some non-white groups that show lower recovery rates are excluded from reporting statistics.[48]

6. **Earlier Detection Providing for longer Survival Rates** - Improvements in technology provide earlier detection, so doctors have gotten quicker to conclude that symptoms might be cancer. However, this early detection has been manipulated over the years to imply longer survival rates, rather than early detection rates.[49]

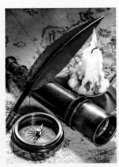

43 Pierce, Tanya Harter. *Outsmart Your Cancer: Alternative Non-Toxic Treatments That Work.* Stateline, NV: Thoughtworks Publishing, 2009 (second edition).
44 Ibid.
45 Ibid.
46 Ibid.
47 Ibid.
48 Ibid.
49 Ibid.

PART V: How Conventional Treatments Have Failed

You don't need to
just SEE your doctor,
you need to BE your doctor.

how cure IS DEFINED

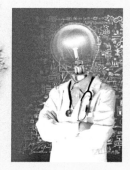

The ACS, NCI, and FDA have all chosen to define cure as alive five years after diagnosis. This official definition does not mean cancer-free, healthy, strong, vigorous, or healed of the disease. To cure actually means to relieve a person of the symptoms of a disease or condition, not necessarily the elimination of the primary causes that continue the recurrences of more cancers and other diseases.

A patient can be diagnosed with cancer, and die five years and one day after the unfortunate diagnosis and receiving ineffective treatments, and they have been classified as cured of the disease according to the current medical authorities. This insight comes from Dr. Ralph W. Moss, PhD. in his book, *The Cancer Industry* (1999). Because of the American Cancer Society's definition of cure, many patients who live five years after their diagnosis are listed as cured - even though they were never cancer-free, still showed evidence of having cancer, progressively lost quality of life, confined to a wheelchair or hospital bed, and even though they actually die from the cancer, they now are statistically listed as cured.

To suggest that these poor unfortunate souls were cured, listed as such on official records, and that these cure rates are now used by the cancer authorities to prove to us their treatments are safe and successful is an outrage and a gross distortion of the real facts and the truth. Yet, that is how we count cancer cures currently in the United States. These are the statistics we are asked to bet on with our faith, hope, energy, money, and our life.

It simply goes without saying that by redefining reality, or the accepted definition of any term, one could prove just about anything. As Mark Twain said, "There are three kinds of lies: lies, damn lies, and statistics."

PART V: How Conventional Treatments Have Failed

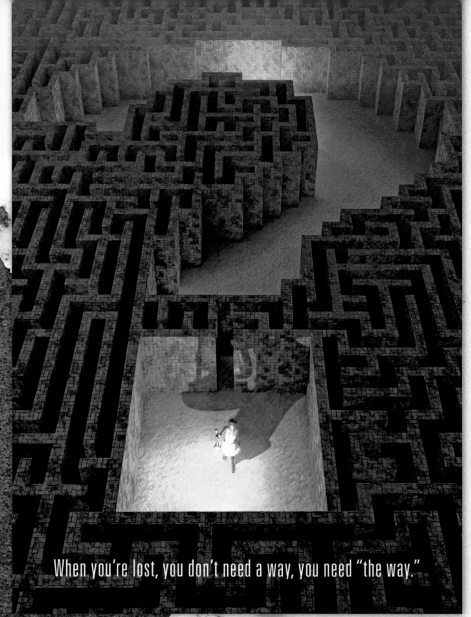

When you're lost, you don't need a way, you need "the way."

EXCERPT FROM CANCERS ANSWERS

VOLUME 1 ✦ PAGE 512
CANCERSANSWERS.ORG

RELATIVE SURVIVAL rate

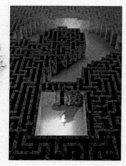

Relative Survival Rate is another *adjustment* to the official cancer cure rate statistics. The thinking, adopted in the early 1980's, goes something like this, "If the person had not died of cancer he might have been run over by a truck, and that must be factored into the equation," according to Dr. Ralph Moss.[50]

Relative Survival Rate is an *official adjustment* that takes into account the expected mortality figures that could be expected in the general population. In effect, it reduces the actual number of cancer deaths statistically and was created to help the cancer authorities claim that the war on cancer was working and being won.

In the previous section on *How Cure is Defined,* we showed how changing the definition of cure improves the cancer survival rate statistics. By changing the definition of survival rate, these statistics are improved even further. Clearly, **these statistical *adjustments* are misleading**, and when the seriously ill are carefully considering their medical options, they tend to rely heavily on the doctor's opinion, these statistics, opinions of family members and friends, and other people in the individual's decision-making process. **By distorting the truth, once again, the cancer authorities are doing a great injustice to the general public and to those most afflicted with catastrophic diagnosis and illness.** Furthermore, these statistical *adjustments* provide cover for the authorities and FDA to continue down the course **many researchers consider being the least effective treatment options for cancer: surgery, chemotherapy and radiation.**

---

[50] Ibid.

PART V: How Conventional Treatments Have Failed

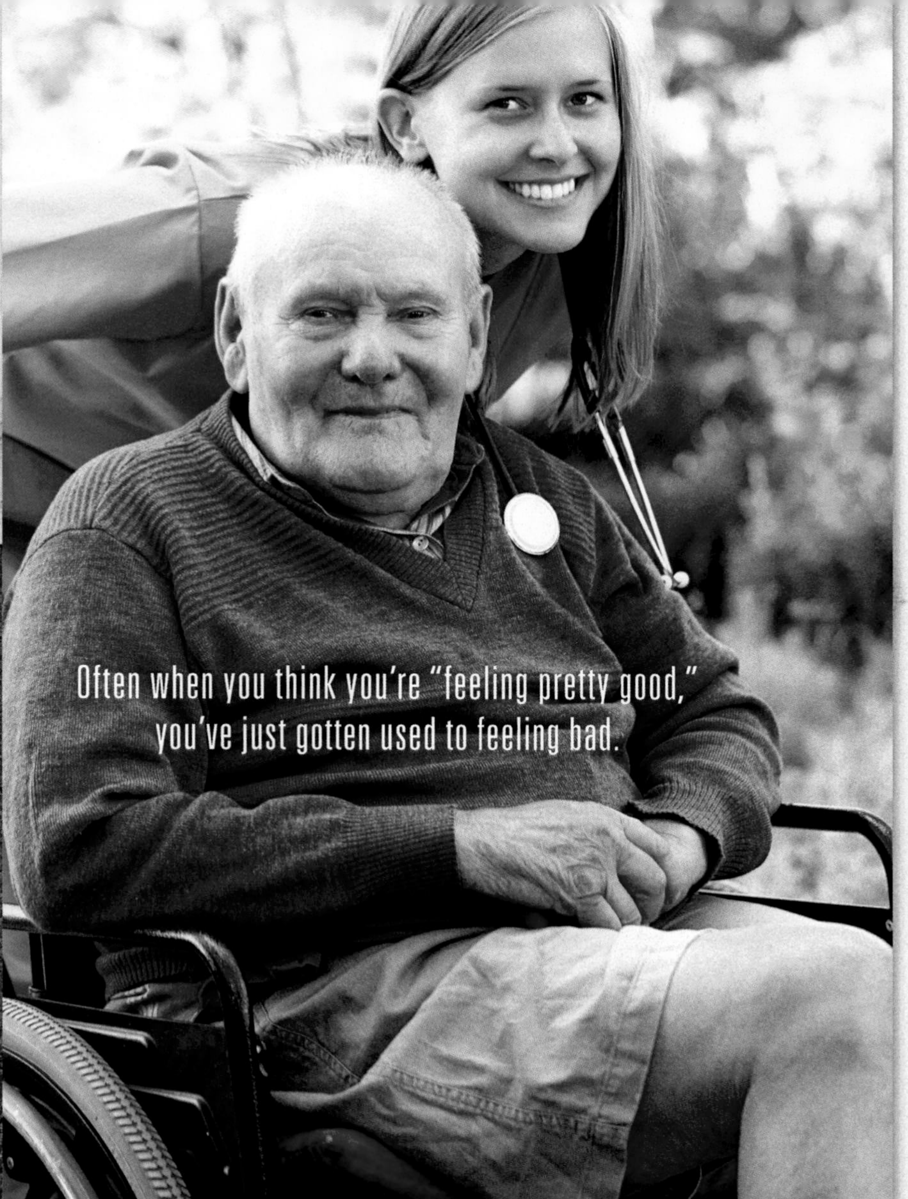

Often when you think you're "feeling pretty good," you've just gotten used to feeling bad.

EXCERPT FROM CANCERS ANSWERS

VOLUME 1 + PAGE 155

CANCERSANSWERS.ORG

patients WHO DIE BEFORE TREATMENT IS COMPLETED

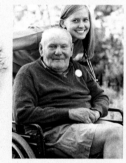 If a cancer patient dies before completing a particular cancer treatment protocol, they are removed from the statistics regarding survival rates. This thinking is based on the presumption that if the patient had lived long enough with their cancer to be treated with surgery, radiation, and/or chemotherapy, they may have survived. Therefore, they must be removed from the survival rate statistics because they did not complete their course of treatment. **This is absurd.** The truth is that the patient died of cancer and the treatments did not save the patient and/or actually contributed to his/her death.

Cancer is particularly insidious because it progresses extremely rapidly in the end stages. *Cancer slowly kills you fast.* It is not unfair to suggest that a particular treatment does not work effectively enough, or fast enough to save a patient, because almost all protocols, be they conventional or alternative, don't do anything about actual causes and have little to no positive affect on actual quality of life conditions of the individual's body. Even though symptoms can be manipulated with medical treatments, long-term survival is substantially reduced and any short-term success mostly comes with a long-term price (short-term success and long-term failure).

The fact that the cancer survival rates are statistically manipulated by eliminating cancer deaths before treatment protocols are completed is nothing less than deceitful. Suggesting that cancer survival rates are better than they are by eliminating cancer deaths before protocol completion is itself misleading and insidious.

If the cancer patient dies of their cancer, most people would conclude that the treatment had failed to save the patient. However, if the patient dies on day 59 of a 60-day protocol, that is not considered a failure? **Death from the disease is not considered a failure of treatment**. Again, by redefining obvious terminology, our cancer success rates are improved statistically (manipulated) so that the cancer authorities can continue to profit and claim a victory in the war on cancer, a war most cancer researchers believe we will never win with such historic conflicts of interest, deceit and abuses.

PART V: How Conventional Treatments Have Failed

Cancer slowly kills you fast.

CANCERS THAT ARE
not life-threatening

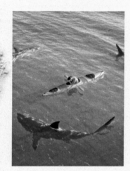

Some cancers are not life-threatening, non-metastasizing, and fairly easily maintained. Many skin cancers, some pre-cancerous breast conditions, and other localized cancers can be successfully treatable. However, including certain conditions in the official cancer survival rate statistics is misleading. According to Dr. Douglas Brodie in his book, *Cancer and Common Sense: Combining Science and Nature to Control Cancer* (1997), "Five year survivals of non-melanoma skin cancers, localized cancers of the cervix, and some other non-spreading cancers detected early in specific sites, have been 'manageable' since the days of Ptolemy."[51]

Other pre-cancerous states such as ductal carcinoma in situ (DCIS) are believed by many medical experts to not even be classified as cancers because they are manageable in the majority of cases. However, almost 30% of all breast cancer diagnoses is DCIS and is included in the life-threatening cancer statistics used here in the U.S. **This fact distorts the true cure and survival rates** of conventional treatment for breast cancer dramatically.

Accidental death is the leading cause of death in the United States up to age 42. The top five accidental deaths include motor vehicle accidents, poisoning, falls, fires, and choking, followed by drowning. Adding non-life threatening conditions to deadly cancer statistics is like adding bike-riding accidents (more than 500,000 emergency room visits per year) to motor vehicle fatalities, which account for more than 40,000 deaths per year. Clearly, **adjusting statistics in this way can substantially skew the success rates of conventional treatments**. The problem is that the **survival rates are not presented accurately or portrayed honestly**. It's hard to understand, until you follow the money, why the cancer authorities, with a true survival rate of only 2 - 3%, wouldn't want to improve the actual rates. If there was a 3% survival rate for skydiving, they would not be allowed to even manufacture parachutes and no one would agree to do it.

[51] Ibid.

PART V: How Conventional Treatments Have Failed

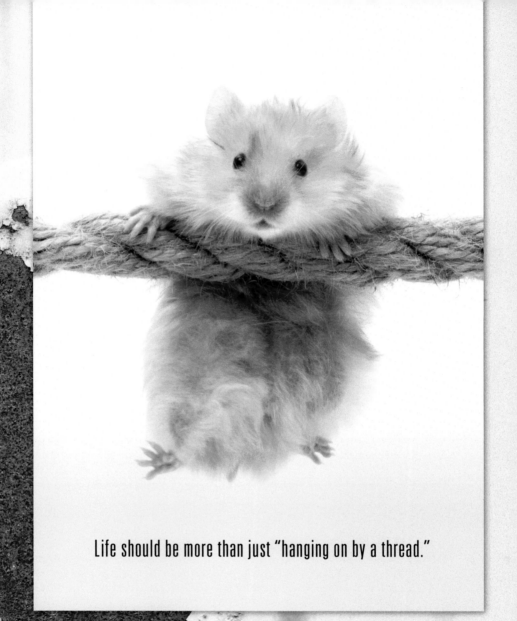

Life should be more than just "hanging on by a thread."

EXCERPT FROM CANCERS ANSWERS

VOLUME 1 + PAGE 532
CANCERSANSWERS.ORG

exclusion OF CERTAIN GROUPS

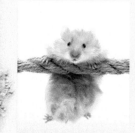

Believe it or not, many cancer statistics include whites-only statistics, and some reports remove lung cancer, America's deadliest cancer, from their statistics completely. How can this possibly be? As it turns out, the National Cancer Institute (NCI) "generally reports whites-only figures," according to the findings of researchers in the New England Journal of Medicine.[52]

"Non-whites are kept in a separate category, not calculated with the main group." Dr. Ralph Moss states that "NCI's solution is to list them in separate (but equal) charts, and then to present the white charts as the norm."[53]

Dr. Moss also says that the NCI has been known to remove lung cancer statistics from overall cancer cure rate statistics. Apparently, lung cancer is seen as different from other cancers by the NCI, using as an excuse its dubious connection to smoking. According to Dr. Marc Micozzi, a prominent and highly regarded researcher at the NCI at that time, in his Monthly Newsletter the *Daily Dispatch*, he says that reports in the largest study ever done on health (1984), including lung cancer show that **only about 10% of life-long smokers ever develop lung cancer**, and that lung cancer occurs to non-smokers in about 1% of the population. How did they get their cancer? It's why, or die!

That same report also shows that smoking less than half a pack a day showed that smoking had virtually no measurable effect on lung cancer, and that pipe or cigar smokers showed better overall health (two pipes or two cigars, or less per day) than the general population. Certainly they are not promoting smoking. However, lung cancer is not primarily caused by smoking alone. The mechanism of action (cause) has not been clearly recognized, identified, or understood. Our treatment of lung cancer is close to non-existent and non-effective, and the cancer authorities have done no serious studies on lung cancer since 1984. Lung cancer is our deadliest cancer and these statistics indicate there are other causes besides smoking. Many researchers believe that the governmental and political agenda is at work here, not to mention all the jobs and profits that could be at stake.

[52] Ibid.
[53] Ibid.

PART V: How Conventional Treatments Have Failed

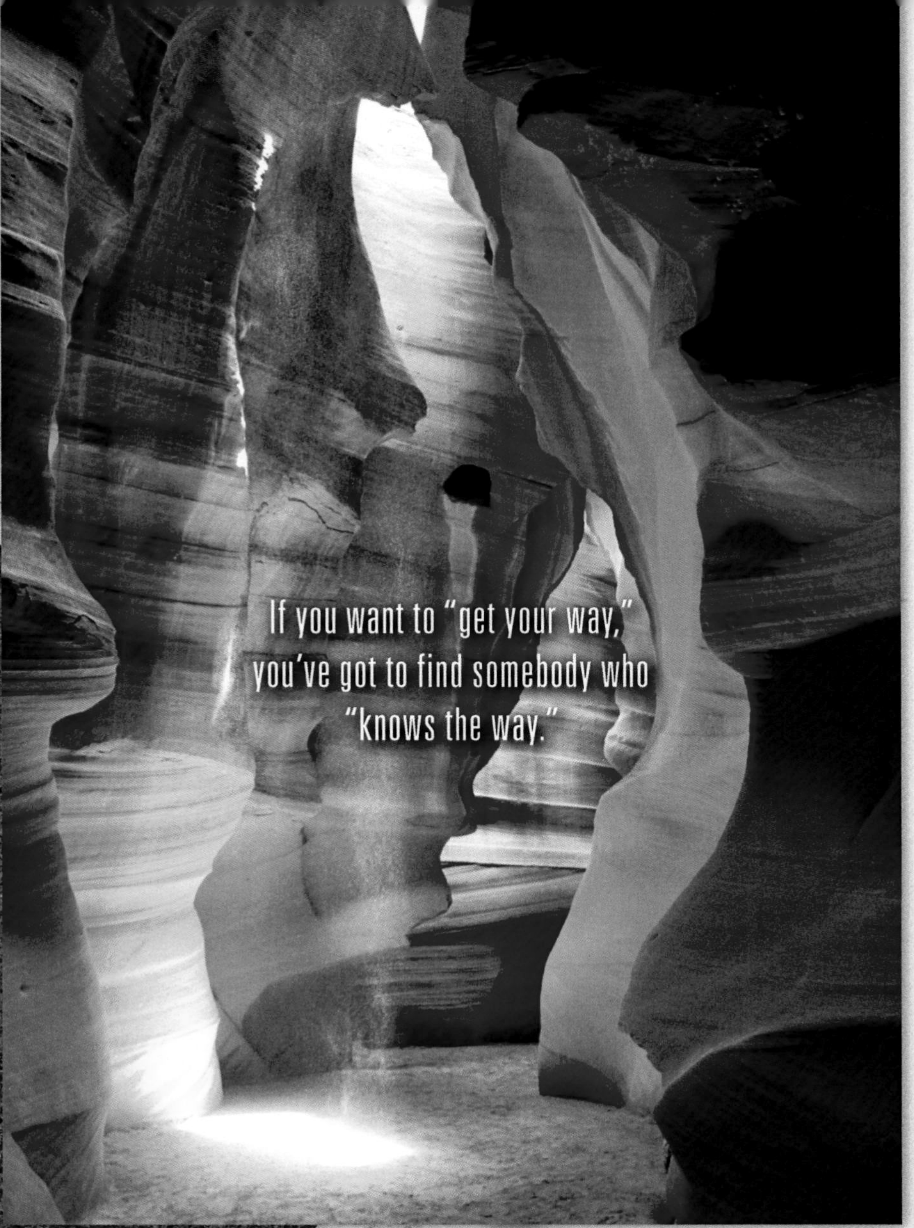

If you want to "get your way,"
you've got to find somebody who
"knows the way."

EXCERPT FROM CANCERS ANSWERS

VOLUME 1 + PAGE 545
CANCERSANSWERS.ORG

exclusionOF CERTAIN GROUPS

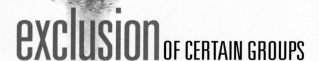

Eliminating lung cancer and non-white cancer deaths from statistics and presenting these statistics as representative of all cancer patients and all life-threatening cancers is not just a case of **biased selection**, but, in fact, a patent falsehood. This practice misleads the public and, more importantly, misleads cancer patients themselves, obstructing vital information and accurate statistics necessary to make an informed decision about their treatment, quality of life and long-term survival potential. Additionally, these inaccurate statistics when presented to patients by their doctors and physicians, whether they know the truth about these statistics or not, is nothing less than a betrayal of our trust in doctors and uninformed confidence, making nearly impossible decisions about cancer treatment, truly impossible.

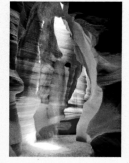

PART V: How Conventional Treatments Have Failed

Fate is a combination of choices.

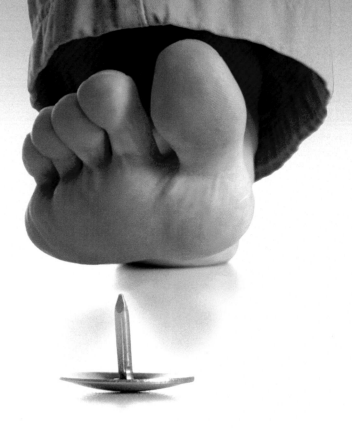

EXCERPT FROM CANCERS ANSWERS

VOLUME 1 ◆ PAGE 557
CANCERSANSWERS.ORG

technology Provides Earlier
Detection Falsely Implying Longer Survival Rates

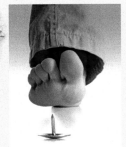

One area where cancer treatment has improved is in its early detection due to improved technology. Doctors can diagnose cancer about six months earlier today, than they could in past years. And that could be a good thing. However, because of the way cure is defined as life or death after five years after diagnosis, we've effectively ONLY improved the statistics by increasing the time frame to the cure deadline by 10%, not actual life expectancy of patients themselves. This would be an actual significant improvement if, in fact, life expectancy was also increased. Unfortunately, this creates a *false perception* engineered by the cancer establishment that is not really true in reality.

The cancer establishment has manipulated the long-term survival rates to look better today than they did years ago, but **NO ACTUAL LONG-TERM SURVIVAL HAS OCCURRED according to most researchers**. This is a statistic, which has improved primarily from manipulation of other statistics and misrepresentation of statistics, but **not in terms of actual life expectancy**, only in terms of these manipulated statistics, which are seriously flawed in the many ways we have discussed. It is important to know what the actual statistics truly are, and what they accurately represent.

We didn't lose the game; we just ran out of time.

- Vince Lombardi

PART V: How Conventional Treatments Have Failed

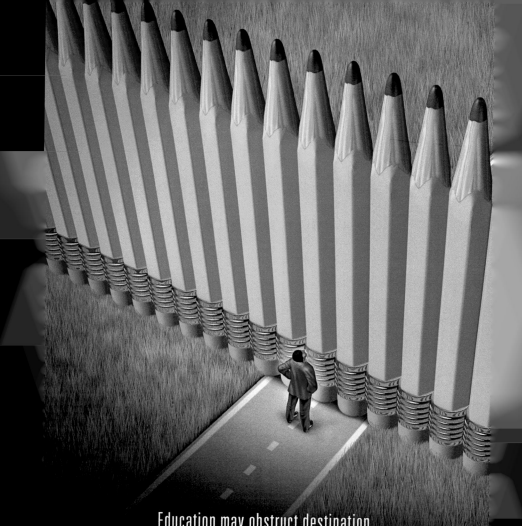

Education may obstruct destination.

EXCERPT FROM CANCERS ANSWERS

VOLUME 1 + PAGE 117

CANCERSANSWERS.ORG

SUMMARY CONCLUSIONS

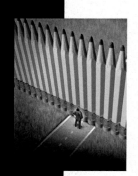

The following facts and descriptions are from the report, their sources footnoted and referenced:

1. Chemotherapy is a poisonous, toxic, carcinogenic (cancer causing) treatment with devastating side effects that can lead to a host of major complications including death.[1] The fact is that most patients treated with chemotherapy die from the chemotherapy before the tumors and cancer could kill them.[2,3]

2. Chemotherapy has no success rate with the major cancers including colon, breast and lung malignancies and only limited success with small tumors that have recently developed. This is a very small fraction of cancers.[4]

3. Shrinking of tumors has no long-term effect on, or correlation to longevity and cancer survival rates.[5]

. . . continued

The least of things with a meaning is worth more in life than the greatest of things without it.
- Carl Jung

[1] Wikipedia. http://en.wikipedia.org/wiki/Chemotherapy.

[2] Cairns, John. "The Treatment of Diseases and the War Against Cancer." *Scientific American* 253:51-9, November 1985.

[3] Moss, Ralph W. *The Cancer Industry*. Page 82. State College, PA, 1999, 2002.

[4] Ibid.

[5] Benson, Jonathan. "Why chemotherapy doesn't work - Cancer tumors confirmed to have stem cells that regenerate tumors." *Natural News.com*, 2012

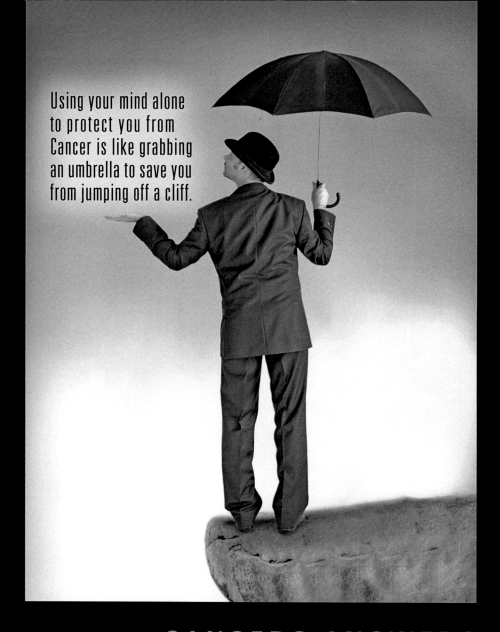

Using your mind alone to protect you from Cancer is like grabbing an umbrella to save you from jumping off a cliff.

EXCERPT FROM CANCERS ANSWERS

VOLUME 1 ✦ PAGE 34

CANCERSANSWERS.ORG

102

SUMMARY CONCLUSIONS

CONTINUED

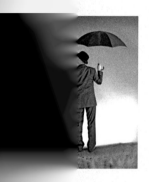

4. The actual 5-year survival rate of adults using chemotherapy is 2.1%, or slightly less than the 5-year survival rate of adults who receive no treatment at all for their cancer.[6]

5. Once the cancer has metastasized, the long-term survival rate for cancer patients using conventional treatment is about 1%.[7]

6. Approximately 5-10% of patients die from leukemia within 10 years of their conventional treatment.[8,9]

7. Most cancer patients in this country die from chemotherapy.[10]

8. Cancer treatments cost about $100,000 - 850,000 per year per patient.[11]

. . . continued

---

[6] Morgan, G., Ward, R., and Barton, M. PubMed.gov. from *Clinical Oncology (R Coll Radioll)* 2004, Dec; 16(8):549-60

[7] Ibid.

[8] Moss, Ralph W. *The Cancer Industry*. Page 82. State College, PA, 1999, 2002.

[9] Cairns, John. "The Treatment of Diseases and the War Against Cancer." *Scientific American* 253:51-9, November 1985.

[10] Lynes, B. *The Healing of Cancer*. "Interview with Allen Levin, MD." Marcus Books, June, 1990.

[11] Micozzi, Marc S. *Insider's Cures*. Baltimore, MA: Insiders-Cures website. 2013.

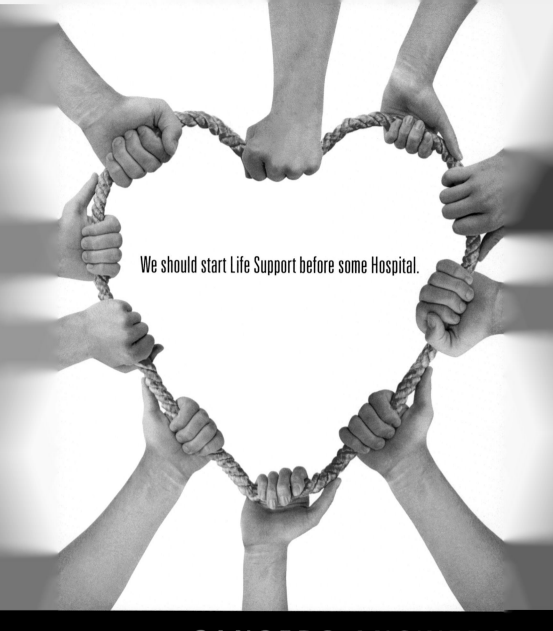

We should start Life Support before some Hospital.

EXCERPT FROM CANCERS ANSWERS

VOLUME 1 + PAGE 556

CANCERSANSWERS.ORG

SUMMARY CONCLUSIONS

CONTINUED

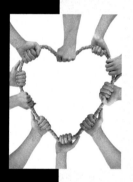

9. 90.6% of oncologists said that chemotherapy was unacceptable for them and their family members in a recent study.[12]

10. Oncologists make 2/3 of their practice revenue from the sale of chemotherapy, which they administer to their patients. This is a massive conflict of interest and likely accounts for 1/3 of cancer patients being treated with chemotherapy by doctors that know in advance the cancers will be unresponsive to the chemotherapy.[13]

11. The claim of cure rates of 40 - 50% is based on flawed methodology on the statistics. The reality is that once the veil is lifted, the actual cancer cure rate is closer to 2 - 3%.[14]

. . . continued

Most people are so afraid of dying they are willing to kill themselves to avoid it.

Battles are not won by trying.

12 Day, Phillip. Cancer: *Why We're Still Dying to Know the Truth.* New York: Credence Publishing, 1999.

13 Abelson, Reed. "Drug Sales Bring Huge Profits, and Scrutiny, to Cancer Doctors." *The New York Times.* New York, January 26, 2003.

14 Pierce, Tanya Harter. *Outsmart Your Cancer: Alternative Non-Toxic Treatments That Work.* Stateline, NV: Thoughtworks Publishing, 2009 (second edition).

We don't know how dirty something is until we try to clean it.

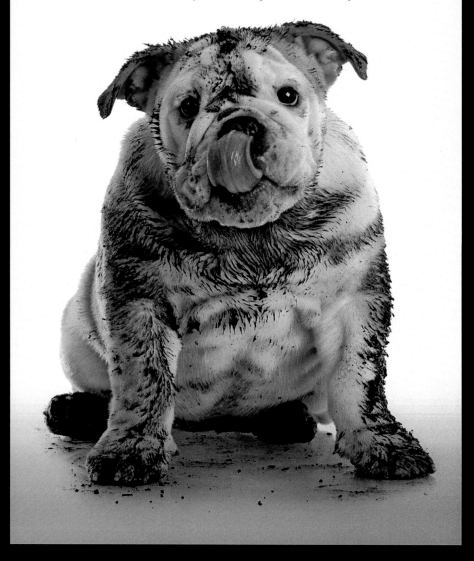

EXCERPT FROM CANCERS ANSWERS

VOLUME 1 ✦ PAGE 378

CANCERSANSWERS.ORG

SUMMARY CONCLUSIONS

&

CONTINUED

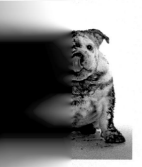

12. The cure statistics quoted by the cancer industry are adjusted to show a more positive result for chemotherapy, as follows:[15]

a How *Cure* is defined - Alive for five (5) years after diagnosis does not mean cancer free, or even good health.

b Relative Survival Rate - The Relative Survival Rate discounts/ reduces the number of cancer deaths by adjusting for patients who may have died by other means, e.g., being run over by a bus.

c Deletion of Patients Who Die Before Treatment is Completed - If the patient dies of cancer before the cancer treatment protocol is completed, he/she is dropped from the cancer death rate statistics.

d Including Non life-threatening Cancer Types - Simple cancers like skin cancers that are easily treated are added to more serious cancer "cure" rates.

e Exclusion of Certain Groups - Some non-white groups that show lower recovery rates are excluded from some reporting statistics.

f Earlier Detection Providing for *Longer* Survival Rates - Improvements in technology provide earlier detection. However, this early detection has been used over the years to imply longer survival rates, rather than early detection rates.

Ten people who speak make more noise than ten thousand who are silent.

\- Napoleon

[15] Pierce, Tanya Harter. Outsmart Your Cancer: *Alternative Non-Toxic Treatments That Work*. Stateline, NV: Thoughtworks Publishing, 2009 (second edition).

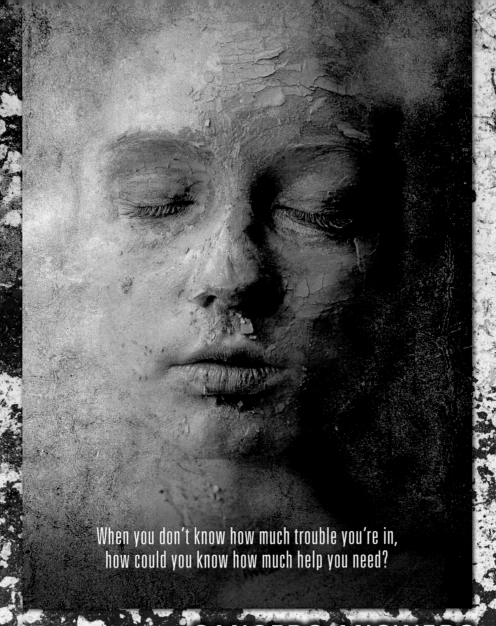

When you don't know how much trouble you're in,
how could you know how much help you need?

EXCERPT FROM **CANCERS ANSWERS**
VOLUME 1 + PAGE 99
CANCERSANSWERS.ORG

So why the obsession with ▪ tumor size?

Well, we can prove (see) that we can shrink tumor size (seeing is believing, right?), but we cannot prove that the survival rate from cancer is any longer today than it was 50 years ago. **The tumor rarely kills the patient; the continuation of the conditions and causes of breeding, feeding, and spreading of the cancer does. The only thing we know for certain is that we are treating the wrong thing!** It's like cutting the tail off the mythical dragon and he just grows a new one. Sound familiar? It's the head that must be killed, not the tail. It's the root of the tree, not the dead leaves on a limb that's the problem. It's the root cause(s) that must be identified and eliminated.

While we need to be focused on strengthening the immune system, we are instead focused on shrinking the tumor, whether the patient survives or not. The fact is that in the war on cancer, a war most researchers believe we have lost, the cancer authorities have little, if anything, to hang their hats on. That's why **they focus on tumor size -- because they can shrink it, whether it stops the cancer, kills the patient, or not. They consider the shrinking of a tumor success long after that patient is dead and hold that out to others as an example as to why they also should do chemotherapy. Yeah, but what about surviving and thriving?**

PART IV: Understanding Conventional Cancer Treatment

71

Every choice you let another make
is your choice.

EXCERPT FROM CANCERS ANSWERS

VOLUME 1 ♦ PAGE 195
CANCERSANSWERS.ORG

references

Day, Phillip. *Cancer: Why We're Still Dying to Know the Truth*. New York: Credence Publishing, 1999.

Douglass, William C., II. *Into the Light*. New York: Rhino Publishing, 2003.

Epstein, Samuel S. The Politics of Cancer. San Francisco: Sierra Book Club, 1978. *Are We Losing The War Against Cancer*? Congressional Record, 1987.

Glade, MJ. "Food, nutrition and the prevention of cancer: a global perspective." *Nutrition:* World Cancer Research Fund (1997), June 15, 1999.

Griffin, G. Edward. *World Without Cancer: The Story of Vitamin B-17.* Thousand Oaks, California: American Media, 1975.

Hoffman, Frederick L. *Cancer and Diet*. Baltimore: Williams and Wilkins Company, 1937.

Huebner, Albert L. "The No-Win War on Cancer." *East West,* December 1987.

Israel, Lucien. *Conquering Cancer*. New York: Random House, 1978.

Lang, Avis. "The Covert War Against Cancer Patients: Notes From the Front." *Townsend Letter for Doctors 66*, January 1989.

Laszlo, John. *Understanding Cancer*. New York: Harper and Row, 1987.

Lynes, B. *The Healing of Cancer*. "Interview with Allen Levin, MD." Marcus Books, June, 1990.

Mendelsohn, Robert. *Dissent in Medicine: Nine Doctors Speak Out*. New York: Contemporary Books, 1985.

Micozzi, Marc S. *Insider's Cures*. Baltimore, MA: Insiders-Cures website. 2013. *Complementary and Integrative Medicine in Cancer Care and Prevention: Foundations and Evidence-Based Interventions*. New York: Springer Publishing Company, 2006. *Fundamentals of Complementary and Alternative Medicine*. New York: Saunders, 2010.

Morgan, G, Ward, R, Barton, M. " The contribution of cytotoxic chemotherapy to 5-year survival in adult malignancies." C*linical Oncology,* December 16, 2004.

Moss, Ralph W. *The Cancer Industry*. State College, PA, 1999, 2002. *Questioning Chemotherapy*. State College, PA: Equinox Press, October 8, 1996.

National Cancer Institute. *Fact Book*. DHEW Publication. Bethesda, MA, 1999. "Radiation Therapy for Cancer." *Fact Sheet*, 2010.

Richards, Dick. *The Topic of Cancer: When the Killing Has to Stop*. New York: Pergamon Press, 1981.

St. John, Tamara. *Defeat Cancer Now: A Nutritional Approach to Wellness for Cancer and Other Diseases*. New York: 48hrbooks.com, 2012. *Cancer Therapy: The Independent Consumer's Guide to Non-Toxic Treatment and Prevention*. State College, PA: Equinox Press, 1996. *Customized Cancer Treatment: How a Powerful Lab Test Predicts Which Drugs Will Work for You-And Which to Avoid*. State College, PA: Equinox Press, 2010. *The Cancer Industry: Unraveling the Politics*. Shreveport, LA: Paragon Press, 1990.

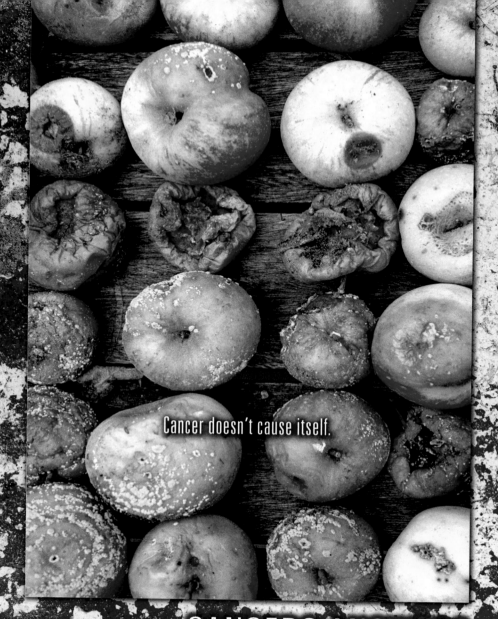

Cancer doesn't cause itself.

EXCERPT FROM CANCERS ANSWERS

VOLUME 1 ✦ PAGE 6

CANCERSANSWERS.ORG

112

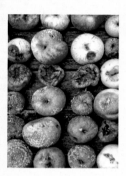

Power up before you power down.

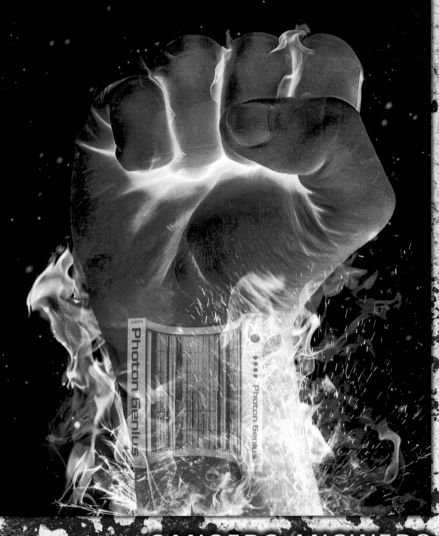